HANDBOOK OF INTERNATIONAL FOOD REGULATORY TOXICOLOGY
Volume 2: Profiles

HANDBOOK OF INTERNATIONAL FOOD REGULATORY TOXICOLOGY
Volume 2: Profiles

Gaston Vettorazzi, M.D., Ph.D.
Scientist, Food Safety Program
World Health Organization, Geneva

and Professor of Experimental Toxicology
University of Milan

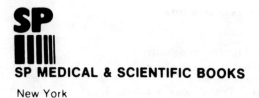

SP MEDICAL & SCIENTIFIC BOOKS
New York

SPECTRUM PUBLICATIONS, INC.
175-20 Wexford Terrace, Jamaica, N.Y. 11432

Library of Congress Cataloging in Publication Data

Vettorazzi, G.
  Handbook of international food regulatory toxicology.

  Includes bibliographical references and index.
    1. Food additives—Toxicology. 2. Pesticide residues in food.
3. Pesticides—Toxicology. 4. Toxicity testing I. Title [DNLM: 1. Food additives—Toxicity—Handbooks. 2. Food analysis—Handbooks. 3. Food contamination—Prevention and control—Handbooks. 4. Pesticide residues—Toxicity—Handbooks.
WA701 V592h]
RA1270.F6V47   615.9′54′028   79-24008
ISBN 0-89335-086-9
ISBN 0-89335-118-0 (V.2)

PREFACE

One of the striking features of our times is the increasing utilization of chemical products in different fields of human activities, as a result of the spectacular progress of chemical research. Our food supply has not been spared from this general trend, however, and chemical substances are being continuously incorporated in foodstuffs. Some of these substances are added to food for technological purposes such as preserving food from bacterial deterioration (antimicrobials), protecting it from oxidative changes (antioxidants), and improving its organoleptic characteristics (sweeteners, flavors, and flavor enhancers), or texture (stabilizers, emulsifiers, colorants). These substances are generally referred to as intentional food additives.

Chemical substances may also be found in food as a result of environmental or accidental contamination. Between these two categories of chemicals, a third class occupies an intermediate position, represented by chemical products utilized to control insect or fungus pests in agriculture and ectoparasites in animal husbandry. These products are currently referred to as pesticides and, due to some of their properties, such as chemical stability associated with scarce hydrosolubility, they may be found as residues in or on food from plant and animal origin. In addition, certain drugs that stimulate growth for accelarating productivity in animals may also be found as residues in edible animal tissues. These substances are referred to as unintentional food additives.

The utilization of additives in human food and animal feed brings about undeniable advantages for society. Similarly, the use of pesticides contributes to the preservation of our food resources and constitutes an important means in the fight against starvation.

However, consideration should be also given to the opposing viewpoint. It is an old notion, which Claude Bernard has repeatedly emphasized, that all chemical substances may evoke toxicological effects if the absorbed dose is sufficiently high and the time of exposure is sufficiently long. There are many examples demonstrating that very small doses which do not show any immediate apparent effect may cause harmful effects if the time of exposure extends over a lifetime of otherwise very long periods. They may cause serious symptoms of intoxication because of cumulative phenomena or they may elicit irreversible carcinogenic effects. The addition of chemical substances to food may thus establish optimal conditions for the manifestation of insidious forms of toxicity called long-term effects.

The possibility of causing long-term toxic effects by the use of food additives (food colors, antimicrobials, antioxidants, etc) has alerted toxicologists to require extensive and strict animal testing prior to utilization of these substances in food, in order to protect the health of the consumer.

In this regard, a pioneering role was played in the fifties at the international level by the European Committee of Chronic Toxicity (Eurotox). Around the same period, the International Union against Cancer was also active in evaluating the carcinogenic risk posed by chemical substances intentionally and unintentionally added to foodstuffs.

The World Health Organization (WHO) could not be indifferent to such an important problem and, since 1954, in collaboration with Food and Agriculture Organization of the United Nations (FAO), it has undertaken studies on the subject. An important decision was reached in September 1955, when a conference that met in Geneva, Switzerland, recommended that the Directors-General of the two organizations convene one or more expert committees, concerned with the technical and administrative aspects of the problem of chemical additives in food. The first meeting of a Joint FAO/WHO Expert Committee on Food Additives (JECFA) was held in Rome in December 1956, the most recent meeting (the 23rd) was held in Geneva in April 1979. A second committee, the Joint FAO/WHO Meeting on Pesticide Residues (JMPR) was initiated in 1963 and met annually thereafter; up to the present this committee held 15 sessions. The JMPR has been entrusted with the evaluation of the possible hazards to man arising from the occurrence of residues of pesticides in food.

After each session, these two committees prepare reports and monographs. The monographs contain summaries of technological, chemical, and toxicological studies which have been used to establish acceptable daily intakes (ADIs) and Maximum Residue Limits (MRLs). These publications have constituted the basis on which national regulatory agencies have formulated food laws for the protection of the consumer. Together with other reports dealing with toxicological methodology, these publications have considerably helped to establish the prestige of both FAO and WHO in the field of food safety.

The methodological approaches and the principles of interpretation of toxicological studies underwent continuous evaluation during the last three decades. In their reports, the JECFA and the JMPR have closely followed up the developments in this field and made recommendations. Unfortunately, their comments and suggestions are scattered over many publications and a systematic assemblage of the major conclusions will certainly facilitate the interested parties to locate significant information.

Dr. Gaston Vettorazzi, a WHO staff member since 1972, who actively participated in the deliberations of both the JECFA and JMPR has undertaken, with the present volume, a systematic collection of toxicological methodology and principles of interpretation of experimental findings. I am pleased to write the foreword to this book, since I have been connected with the activities of these two international committees since their outset.

In the last paragraph of his introduction, the author expressed the hope that his work would be of help to all those engaged in research and work in the field of food additives, food contaminants, and pesticides.

I don't think I am biased by my friendship with him when I say that his hope is sure to be fulfilled. He has succeeded in the task he set himself to do. His book meets a real international need and should occupy a place of honor in the book-shelves not only of toxicologists, but also in that of medical doctors, food hygienists, food technologists, agronomists, administrators, food regulatory personnel, as well as industrialists and consumer advocates.

Professor Rene Truhaut
Professor of Toxicology
Member of the "Institut de France"
(Academy of Science)

Contents

INTRODUCTION

Food colorants belong to an important class of food additives. The importance of this class is due to its wide use by the food processors, and is affected by the regulatory efforts carried out in many forums, and recent controversies among consumers, regulatory/experimental toxicologists, and industry.

The practice of coloring foods dates far back in history. However, concerns over the safety of this practice are relatively recent. The introduction of synthetic dyestuffs on the market and the increasing extent to which they were being used in or on food products determined the issuance of many specific laws in many nations at the beginning of this century. Legal measures ranged from absolute prohibition of the use of any color in food, to practically unlimited use of all colorants but a few. Between these two extremes were prohibition of a number of specific dyes and limitation of their use to designated legitimate applications. These prohibitions and limitations represented the initiation of registration programs which, among other regulations, required (and still do) that the manufacturer/user submit proofs of safety to government regulatory officials.

Today, food regulatory toxicology is an established activity exercised by government authorities in many parts of the globe. It is considered a technical specialty aimed at providing the scientific basis for regulation and legal action. When related to food colorants, the major task of regulatory toxicologists consists of defining, whenever possible, predictably safe levels of food colorants to which consumers may be exposed over long periods of time, without appreciable risk to their health. In carrying out his task, the regulatory toxicologist relies upon two main elements: a) an adequate and reliable supply of toxicolgical information; and b) an independent and unbiased expert judgment. The whole process is generally defined as toxicological evaluation of a food colorant.

Today, toxicity, hazard, and safety of a food colorant are largely assessed by utilizing the predictive tools of traditional toxicology that were adapted and expanded to fields other than those of undesirable effects from therapeutic agents and occupational exposure. A complete array of scientific contributions is available from the published and

1

unpublished literature concerning methodologies, principles of interpretation of experimental and epidemiological findings, the validity of
animal experimentation for the prediction of safe levels for man, and
the validity of scientific judgment in the evaluation of safety for man.

It should be recognized that the most uncertain aspect in safety
evaluations is the relevance of animal data to man. This uncertainty
originates not only from the problem of differences of species, but
also, and principally, from the very nature of the type of safety index that one wishes to derive from the maximum daily dose of a chemical
fed continually to an appropriate animal species without ill-effect.
Extrapolation to man from no-effect doses that have been established
in animal models is based on a generally agreed assumption that if a
particular effect is observed in several animal species, the possibility
may exist that the same effect will also be observed in man. At least,
this possibility should not be ruled out without sound and specific
reasons. The choice, however, of a most pertinent criterion of toxicity
for a specific compound could be the subject of considerable dispute
among experts.

With regard to experimental evidence of carcinogenicity in experimental animals, many national and international agencies conform to
the concept of maximum safety when dealing with food colorants. Consequently, the value of experimental results in animals in order to
predict a similar effect in man, has been, for the most part, accepted
as valid. It should, nevertheless, be recognized that no adequate criteria are presently available to interpret experimental data on carcinogenicity directly, in terms of potential to humans.

Apart from many national agencies, there are three international
groups that are actively engaged in the evaluation process of the toxicity of food colorants at the present time. In chronological order of
established activity, the first is the Joint FAO/WHO Expert Committee
on Food Additives, which has been carrying out toxicological assess-
ments of food additives, including food colorants, since 1956. This
committee formulates toxicological decisions and issues recommendations in this regard to all member countries of the World Health Organization and the Food and Agriculture Organization of the United Nations. The second group is the IARC (International Agency for Research
on Cancer) Working Group on the Evaluation of the Carcinogenic Risk of
Chemicals to Man, which began its activities in 1971. This group aims
at assembling, documenting, and evaluating scientific data on chemicals
in general, in term of their carcinogenic potential; on several occa-
sions it has examined data on food colorants. The third group is the
Scientific Committee for Food of the Commission of the European Communities, which was established in 1974 to give advice on any problem
relating to the protection of the health and safety of persons arising
from the consumption of food, and, in particular, the composition of
food additives and other processing aids, as well as the presence of
contaminants. The opinions of this committee are submitted to the Commission of the European Communities and, as a rule, are published.

This book brings together, in a systematic manner, the decisions/
recommendations of the above groups, as well as their main comments on
the toxicity of as many food colorants as available. The core of the
volume consists of toxicity profiles aimed at providing a ready indication of the major toxicological features of the compound, as well as
other important aspects related to the safety of the compound, and to
call the attention of the reader to available sources of references if
an examination in depth is desired.

These reference sources are organized in several ways, in tables, for ready consultation and location. Table III reports, in tabular form, references available on food colorants mentioned in the text. While this table has been carefully designed and completed, it is possible that some omissions might be found, since data which have been found adequate for regulatory purposes have been included primarily.

It is hoped that this work will be of assistance to individuals or groups involved in the toxicological assessment of food colorants for regulatory purposes or otherwise.

Chapter 1

General Principles in the Toxicological Evaluation of Food Colorants

Food colorants should be considered to be food additives and, consequently, be subjected to the general principles governing the use of food additives (1) and to the procedures for testing their safety (2, 3,4).

1. TECHNOLOGICAL JUSTIFICATION FOR COLORANTS IN FOOD

The use of food colorants is technologically justified when the benefit to the consumer is involved. Thus, maintenance of the nutritional quality of a food and making foods attractive to the consumer could represent two justifications of the intentional addition of colorants to food (5).

It is desirable, in all circumstances, to maintain the nutritional quality of foods; but this is especially important in countries in which the supply of essential nutrients in the usual diet is marginal or deficient. Any nutritional losses may then become serious; and it is particularly necessary to avoid losses of the less stable vitamins. A typical example of the use of an additive in checking such losses is the addition of an antioxidant to edible fats which contain substantial amounts of beta-carotene or vitamin A, destruction of which may be accelerated by the onset of rancidity during storage. In certain circumstances, the nutritional value of a food may be enhanced incidentally by the use of additives. Thus, ascorbic acid, when employed as an antioxidant, will increase the antiscorbutic value of foods, such as fruit products, to which it is added, while the coloring of margarine with beta-carotene will enhance its vitamin A activity (6).

Non-nutritive additives used to increase the appeal of a food to the consumer are, chiefly, colors, flavoring agents, emulsifying, stabilizing and thickening agents, bleaching agents, and clarifiers. The value of color in food products lies mainly in the fact that the interest of consumers in a food may decrease if it does not have the color to which they have become accustomed. Typical instances are manufactured dairy products, such as butter and cheese, the natural color of which may vary from season to season; canned and pulped fruits and vegetables, which have lost some of their original color during the processing necessary for their preservation; sugar confectionery; and beverages.

The desire that certain foods be without color, and the preference for a certain consistency in a food or beverage, a clear beverage, or other special properties in foods, has led to the use of other additives such as bleaching agents, thickeners, and clarifiers.

Certain plant, fish, and animal products formerly used largely as animal food are increasingly being used as human food. In several instances, this has been made possible through the application of food additives such as flavors, colors, and agents which improve texture.

Attention must be drawn to the fact that processing practices made possible by the use of additives which increase the appeal of food to consumers should not lead to their deception. Adequate labeling of food products will help to prevent such deception (7).

The importance of food additives has been stressed in relation to the food-population equation. The continuing increase in the world population without a comparable increase in the available amount of conventional foodstuff must stimulate further efforts to develop new sources of food. In addition to ensuring the safety of these new foods, there is also a need to ensure their palatability and acceptability to consumers; thus, food additives will be required for the purpose of preserving, texturizing, flavoring, and coloring them (8).

2. SAFETY FOR USE OF FOOD COLORANTS

The most important factor for the acceptance of a substance as a food additive is, however, the establishment of its safety in use. This implies that an adequate toxicological evaluation has to be made (9). While it is impossible to establish absolute proof of the non-toxicity of a specified use of an additive for all human beings under all conditions, critically designed animal tests of the physiological, pharmacological, and biochemical behavior of the proposed food additive can provide a reasonable basis for evaluating the safety of its use at a specified level of intake. Any decision to use an intentional additive must be based on the considered judgment of properly qualified scientists that the intake of the additive will be substantially below any level which could be harmful to consumers. The decision as to a safe level should be based on knowledge of the maximum dietary level that does not produce an unfavorable response in test animals, of the severity and type of response in animals above that level, and of the estimated potential intake of the additive (10).

In applying these concepts to the use of food colorants, it has been observed that, while there are cases in which the use of these additives is justified, the best method for regulation is the establishment of a list of permitted colorants which have been adequately tested by animal experimentation. There is agreement that colorants that produce cancer on oral administration must be eliminated from these lists. There are, however, some colorants which do not produce cancer in animal feeding tests but which, on injection, produce a significant number of sarcomas at the site of injection. In some countries, induction of such sarcomas is considered sufficient to indicate that a substance cannot be regarded as safe for man, and it is considered prudent to reject such substances for use in food until more proof of safety is available. In any case, the use of food colorants which have not been sufficiently tested is undesirable--particularly those which are known to be carcinogenic, such as auramine O, and tetramethyl diamino diphenyl cetonimine hydrochloride, etc.

Since the components (e.g. beta-naphthylamine in yellow OB and AB) or other impurities present in food colorants may be carcinogenic, it is particularly important that rigid chemical specifications be established and maintained for all food colorants. In all cases, the potential risks should be considered in relation to the advantages of their use (11).

3. TOXICOLOGICAL EVALUATION OF FOOD COLORANTS

The toxicological decisions are reached solely on the basis of toxicological and related information. Questions concerning the need for food colorants or their technical suitability are the province of other groups--at the international level, the Codex Alimentarius Committee on Food Additives (12).

3.1 Specifications for identity and purity

3.1.1 Natural food colorants

Natural food colorants have been used over a long period of time and have often been accepted for use in foods without supporting toxicological evidence in much the same manner as vegetables and cereal products. The lack of published information relating to adequate identification and chemical composition represents a serious problem. Natural colorants may be available in different forms; in the case of botanical products, both the powdered plant and the extract of the powdered plant have been used as coloring agents for many years. Also, because of differences in soil, climatic conditions, age of plant, and time of harvest, the nature and proportions of the colored and other components of the same species of the same plant may vary widely. Such products may contain a large percentage of substances which have not been defined. Morphological and histological examination of such botanicals has been used for a long time for the identification and quality evaluation of these materials, but the information obtained in this way is inadequate.

For certain products of other than plant origin--for example, natural and synthetic ultramarines, cochineal, and caramel--similar problems of chemical identification have been encountered.

It is essential that methods of analysis, including adequate identification and quality data, should be available whenever any toxicological evaluation of coloring matters of natural origin (13) is undertaken.

Some of the natural food colorants are marketed as dried natural products. Examples are saffron, turmeric, paprika, and dried tagetes meal. In general, these products are not well characterized. Furthermore, insufficient information is available concerning their composition, purity, and use levels. Natural colorants are also sold as extracts. Examples of this type are cochineal extracts, tagetes extracts, and the anthocyanin color in grape-skin extract. The gaps in information concerning natural color extracts are essentially the same as those for the dried natural products.

Oleoresins are another type of natural food colorant. They are obtained by extraction of the coloring principle from the natural product and evaporation of the solvent. Examples of such products are turmeric oleoresin, paprika oleoresin, and corn endosperm oil. The same uncertainties pertain to this type of colorant as to the dried natural colors. In addition, information is lacking concerning the composition of products obtained by extraction of the same natural product with different solvents.

When a food colorant is isolated from natural sources, information
concerning the composition of the coloring product is generally deficient
as compared to that available for synthetic colors. In addition, microbiological specifications are necessary for the colorant isolated from
natural sources. The lack of assurance of reproducible composition of
natural food colorants makes their toxicological evaluation a difficult
task (14).

3.1.2 Synthetic organic food colorants

Identification of dyes is a difficult task, particularly in the case
of the water-soluble sulfonated dyes. Dyes in commerce may be diluted
for convenience of use and other reasons; to specify limits of purity
for the large number of such mixtures marketed has not been attempted.
However, any synthetic organic food colorant should meet adequate specification requirements. Furthermore, specifications for colors synthesized from non-sulfonated aromatic amines should limit such impurities
to not more than 0.02%, and it should be used as starting materials in
to not more than 0.02%, and it should be emphasized that under no circumstances may known carcinogenic amines be used as starting materials in
the production of food colorants. In addition, the availability of substances as reference materials for the synthetic organic food colorants
is essential for their identification and assay (15).

3.2 Toxicological data required for adequate
toxicological evaluation

The fundamental principles on which the evaluation of the acceptability of food additives should be based have been laid down in references 2,3,4,16,17, and 18, and extensively reviewed in reference 19.

In applying these principles to the evaluation of food colorants,
it should be taken into consideration that the use of this class of
food additives is considered by many to be unnecessary (20). As stated
above, while questions of need and technical suitability of food colorants are not in the direct domain of toxicological evaluations, it is,
however, felt that there should be insistence on the fulfillment of the
complete requirements deemed necessary for reliable evaluation (20). It
is useful to list here the main headings under which information should
be available. Apart from chemical and physical specifications dealt
with in section 3.1, information on acute toxicity (21) short-term
toxicity (22) long-term toxicity (23), carcinogenicity studies (24) and
metabolic studies (25,26) is necessary.

In evaluating food colorants, the main emphasis must be placed on
studies of metabolism and long-term toxicity. In the past, many investigations of a long-term nature were tests for carcinogenicity. Often,
the number of animals employed was small and comparisons with control
groups were not made. Many of the toxicological reports contained no
mention of the majority of the observations considered to be an essential
part of long-term toxicity studies. The criteria for long-term studies
that are especially relevant in the case of food colorants are: (a)
growth curves and associated data (23), (b) studies of haemopoietic
function (27), (c) studies of hepatic and renal function, and, where
indicated, the function of other organs (27), (d) organ weights at
autopsy (27) and (e) histopathological investigations (28). The effects
on reproduction and the fetus need to be studied (29).

It should be added that, even when such studies are carried out
in adequate detail, the final reports are often not presented in a form
that permits independent assessment of the validity of the conclusions
reached. Statistical treatment of the results is also often lacking. It

must be stressed that a reliable evaluation can be reached only if detailed information is available concerning the experimental results (30).

A substantial proportion of the available information is found only in unpublished reports. In the past, this has been attributed in part to the lack of suitable media for the publication of results in this field. This situation has now been remedied by the foundation of specialized scientific periodicals.* One of them even undertakes to summarize unpublished data, to submit the summary to the authors for approval, and to assure prompt publication. In view of these circumstances, it may, in the future, be undesirable to assess safety aspects solely on the basis of unpublished work (27).

With regard to the number of animal species, at least two species, one of them a non-rodent, should be used (2,27) in the case of short-term toxicity studies. In the case of long-term toxicity studies, the use of at least two animal species, in tests extending over the major part of the life-span, is recommended (2,27).

For the evaluation of carcinogenic hazard, a life-span feeding study in two animal species (e.g. rats and mice) is recommended as a minimum safeguard (31,32). If these recommendations are followed along the lines recommended in reference 2, both toxicity and carcinogenicity can be assessed in the same study.

The necessity of metabolic studies for purposes of evaluation has been very clearly stated (26,33). In the past, some food additives have been considered acceptable in the absence of adequate information on metabolism. For food colorants, however, there must be insistence on a knowledge of metabolism, since many of these compounds, by their chemical nature, are liable to give rise to potentially toxic degradation products, either by the action of intestinal microorganisms or by metabolic transformation within the body (31).

3.2.1 Natural food colorants

Naturalness per se does not assure safety (34). For purposes of toxicological evaluation, natural food colorants should be considered as falling within three main groups:

a) A colorant isolated in a chemically unmodified form from a recognized foodstuff and used in the foodstuff from which it is extracted at levels normally found in that food. This product could be accepted in the same manner as the food itself, with no requirement for toxicological data.

b) A colorant isolated in a chemically unmodified form from a recognized foodstuff but used at levels in excess of those normally found in that food or used in foods other than those from which it is extracted. This product might require the toxicological data usually demanded to assess the toxicity of synthetic colorants.

c) A colorant isolated from a food source that is chemically modified during its production or a natural colorant isolated from a non-food source. These products would also require a toxicological evaluation similar to that carried out for a synthetic colorant. Furthermore, natural colorants may be reproduced by chemical synthesis. "Nature-identical" colorants produced by chemical synthesis may contain impurities warranting toxicological evaluation similar to those required for a synthetically produced food colorant (35).

---

*E.g. Toxicology and Applied Pharmacology; Food and Cosmetic Toxicology.

3.2.2 Synthetic organic food colorants

The minimum data required for the toxicological evaluation of synthetic organic food colorants are the following:

a) metabolism studies in several species, preferably including man; these studies should include absorption, distribution, biotransformation, and elimination; and an attempt should be made to identify the metabolic products in each of these steps;
b) short-term feeding studies in a non-rodent mammalian species;
c) multigeneration reproduction/teratogenicity studies;
d) long-term carcinogenicity/toxicity studies in two animal species.

Furthermore, recent advances in analytical chemistry, particularly in high-pressure liquid chromatography, would enable the chemical composition of food colorants to be determined more precisely. Together with the technological advances in the manufacture of food colorants, this new technological ability would permit the formulation of more refined chemical specifications for identity and purity, as well as level of undesirable substances, whenever such specifications were requested (36).

4. CLASSIFICATION OF FOOD COLORANTS IN ACCORDANCE WITH THEIR TOXICOLOGICAL EVALUATION

In the past, food colorants were separated into several categories according to their toxicological evaluation and the availability of data on toxicology and other aspects. While this classification can be, at present, considered outdated for some of the compounds, it can still retain some validity. The following categories have been laid down in reference 37:

Category A: This category comprises compounds for which it was possible to establish an acceptable daily intake for man (ADI). While stated that food colorants included in this category could be acceptable for use in food, it was, however, observed that their inclusion should not be interpreted as signifying that further research concerning them was unnecessary. More work was called for, especially in view of the possibility that new advances in science might provide more delicate and accurate means of toxicological assessment.

Category B: In this category are those food colorants for which the available data were not entirely sufficient to meet the requirements for inclusion in Category A.

Category C.I: In this category are compounds for which the available data were inadequate for safety assessment, but for which a substantial amount of detailed information was available concerning results of long-term tests.

Category C.II: This category includes compounds for which the available data were inadequate for safety assessment, and for which virtually no information on long-term toxicity was available. Long-term tests for carcinogenicity unaccompanied by long-term toxicity studies were considered as falling within this category.

Category C.III: In this category are listed those compounds for
which the available data were inadequate for safety assessment, but indicated the possibility of harmful effects.

Category D: This category contains compounds for which virtually
no toxicological data were available.

Category E: Within this category falls those compounds which were
found to be harmful and which should not be used in food.

REFERENCES

1. WHO/FAO. General principles governing the use of food additives.
First report. FAO Nutrition Meetings Report Series, No. 15; Wld.
Hlth. Org. Techn. Rep. Ser., No. 129, 1957.
2. WHO/FAO. Procedures for the testing of intentional food additives
to establish their safety for use. Second report. FAO Nutrition
Meetings Report Series, No. 17; Wld. Hlth. Org. Techn. Rep. Ser.,
No. 144, 1958.
3. WHO/FAO. Evaluation of the carcinogenic hazards of food additives.
Fifth report. FAO Nutrition Meetings Report Series, No. 29; Wld.
Hlth. Org. Techn. Rep. Ser., No. 220, 1961.
4. WHO. Procedures for investigating intentional and unintentional food
additives. Report of a WHO Scientific Group. Wld. Hlth. Org. Techn.
Rep. Ser., No. 348, 1967.
5. WHO/FAO (1957), pp. 5-6.
6. Ibid., p. 5.
7. Ibid., p. 6.
8. WHO/FAO, Evaluation of Certain additives. Some food colours, thickening agents, smoke condensates, and certain other substances. Nineteenth report. FAO Nutrition Meetings Report Series, No. 55; Wld.
Hlth. Org. Techn. Rep. Ser., No. 576, p. 6, 1975.
9. WHO/FAO, Toxicological evaluation of certain food additives with a
review of general principles and specifications. Seventeenth report. FAO Nutrition Meetings Report Series, No. 53; Wld. Hlth. Org.
Techn. Rep. Ser., No. 539, 1974, p. 6.
10. WHO/FAO (1957), p. 8.
11. WHO/FAO (1961), p. 25.
12. WHO/FAO, Specifications for the identity and purity of food additives and their toxicological evaluation: food colours and some
antibicrobials and antioxidants. Eighth report. FAO Nutrition Meetings Report Series, No. 38; Wld. Hlth. Org. Techn. Rep. Ser., No.
309, p. 11, 1965.
13. WHO/FAO (1965), pp. 9-10.
14. WHO/FAO, Evaluation of certain food additives. Twenty-first report.
FAO Food and Nutrition Series, No. 8; Wld. Hlth. Org. Techn. Rep.
Ser., No. 617, pp. -7, 1978.
15. WHO/FAO (1965), p. 10.
16. WHO/FAO, Evaluation of the toxicity of a number of antimicrobials
and antioxidants. Sixth report. FAO Nutrition Meetings Report Series,
No. 31, Wld. Hlth. Org. Techn. Rep. Ser., No. 228, 1962.
17. WHO/FAO, Specifications for identity and purity of food additives
and their toxicological evaluation: emulsifiers, stabilizers,
bleaching and maturing agents. Seventh report. FAO Nutrition Meetings Report Series, No. 35; Wld. Hlth. Org. Techn. Rep. Ser., No.
281, 1964.
18. WHO/FAO (1974).

19. Vettorazzi, G. Handbook of International Food Regulatory Toxicology:
    General Principles, Testing Procedures, and Principles of Interpre-
    tation of Experimental Findings. Elsevier/North Holland Biomedical
    Press B.V. (in publication)
20. WHO/FAO (1965), p. 11.
21. WHO/FAO (1958), p. 9.
22. Ibido., p. 10.
23. Ibid., pp. 11-12.
24. WHO/FAO (1961), pp. 8-14 and 22-23.
25. WHO/FAO (1958), pp. 13-14.
26. WHO/FAO (1962), p. 8.
27. WHO/FAO (1965), p. 12.
28. WHO/FAO (1961), pp. 15-16.
29. WHO/FAO (1958), p. 12.
30. WHO/FAO (1961), p. 33.
31. WHO/FAO (1965), p. 13.
32. WHO/FAO (1961), p. 22.
33. WHO/FAO (1958), p. 33.
34. WHO/FAO (1978).
35. Ibid., p. 7.
36. Ibid., p. 7-8.
37. WHO/FAO (1965), p. 14.

Chapter 2

Toxicological Profiles of Food Colorants

ACID FUCHSINE FE

This triarylmethane compound is found as a mixture of the sodium and ammonium salts of the disulfonic and trisulfonic acids of pararosaniline and rosaniline. This compound has been classified as a color for which the available toxicological data are inadequate for evaluation, and for which virtually no information on long-term toxicity is available (1). The toxicological evidence on which this decision was based is partially found in references 2 and 3.

The oral LD_{50} in the mouse was found to be 1 g/kg bw. Intravenous injection of 0.2 mMol/kg bw in dogs induced vomiting. The color was included in the diet of five male and five female rats at a level of 4 percent for periods up to 18 months; and the animals were observed for up to 20 months. No tumors were observed. Reference to these studies can be found in Table III.

Specifications for identity and purity were prepared, but since no toxicological data on long-term toxicity were available, no toxicological evaluation on this color was carried out (3).

Two reviews on specifications of this compound (3,4) are available, although no review of its toxicity is available.

ACRIDINE ORANGE

This acridine compound has been used to color fats, oils, and waxes bright orange (5). It has been classified as a color for which virtually no toxicological data are available (6), and, consequently, for which no toxicological evaluation has been carried out.

In a subsequent evaluation of the carcinogenic risk of this compound, it has been observed that acridine orange has been tested in mice by skin application; in mice and rats by repeated subcutaneous injection, and in mice by single intraperitoneal injection, followed by skin application of croton oil. The available data were insufficient for an evaluation of the carcinogenicity of this compound to be made (7).

One review on the toxicology of this compound (8) and one on its specifications (9) are available.

ALKALI BLUE

This triarylmethane compound is found as a mixture of the sodium salt of triphenylpararosaniline monosulfonic acid and diphenylrosaniline monosulfonic acid; an example of the latter being the sodium salt of alpha-(4-amino-m-tolyl)-alpha-(p-anilinophenyl)-alpha-hydroxy-p-toluidino benzenesulfonic acid. This compound has been classified as a color for which the available toxicological data are inadequate for evaluation, and for which no information on long-term toxicity is available (1). The toxicological evidence on which this decision was based is found in reference 10.

The oral LD_{50} in the mouse was found to be 9000 mg/kg bw. Twenty rats (10 males and 10 females) were given 10,000 ppm of this color in their diet for 90 days, and compared with a control group. Growth, blood, and urine composition were normal. No histological abnormalities were found in the heart, lung, liver, kidney, or spleen of animals sacrificed six and 14 days after the administration of the color had been stopped. Reference to these studies can be found in Table III.

No review on the toxicologicy of this compound is available but one review on its specifications (11) is.

ALKANET/ALKANNIN

These natural red colors belong to the naphthaquinone chemical class. Alkanet is obtained from the roots of <u>Alkanna tinctoria Tausch</u> (<u>Anchusa tinctoria Lam.</u>) and <u>Lawsonia alba Lam</u>, by extraction with petroleum ether. The coloring principle is alkannin.

Alkanet is a dark red, greenish-reflecting, amorphous powder with a slight acid reaction. It is fat soluble.

Alkannin forms red-brown needles with a coppery luster. It is almost insoluble in water; and is soluble in ethanol, ether, and vegetable oils (12,13).

These colors were not evaluated because of the lack of toxicological information and the lack of knowledge of composition, the variation in composition according to the source, and the method of preparation employed (14). Furthermore, no evidence was available that these substances are found in food commodities moving in international trade(15).

Experiments on rats and mice are available for oral acute toxicity of alkannin. LD_{50} for male mice has been found to be 2.8 g/kg bw and 3.3 g/kg bw for female mice; LD_{50} for rats is above 1 g/kg bw. Alkannin causes diarrhea in male mice in doses above 1.4g/kg bw and in female mice above 1.8 g/kg bw; in rats after doses above 1g/kg bw. Up to 1.4g/kg bw, alkannin does not cause Heinz bodies in mice; it is excreted in the feces, urine, and probably also through the skin; it is deposited in the adipose tissue. The period of lethal outcome of alkannin intoxication is six days; the cause being liver damage.

Alkannin isolated from Radix alkannae tinct. L. Tausch, was used in a 20-week feeding trial in mice, and was added to the diet at a 1 percent level. It caused no changes in body weight or Heinz bodies; and no changes in blood chemistry or morphological alterations were observed in most important organs examined. The dye is excreted in urine and did not accumulate in abdominal fat tissues. Reference to these studies can be found in Table III.

Alkanet was listed among colors for which an acceptable daily intake for man (ADI) could not be established and those which are not toxicologically acceptable for use in food by the Scientific Committee for Food of the Commission of the European Communities (76).

No reviews on the toxicology of these compounds are available. Specifications published in reference 12 were later revoked (16).

ALLURA RED AC

This monoazo color is formed by coupling diazotized 5-amino-4-methoxy-2-toluene sulfonic acid to 6-hydroxy-2-naphthalene sulfonic acid. It was developed for use as a certifiable color in 1967.

Orally administered to experimental animals, this color is rapidly absorbed, as evidenced by coloration of eyes and skin within two hours after intubation of 5 g into dogs. In rats, 71 percent of the color appears to be metabolized, but no metabolites have been identified either in urine or feces. It is suggested that azo reduction by gut flora will form principally 2-methoxy-5-methyl aniline-4-sulfonic acid (cresidine-4-sulfonic acid and 1-amino-2-napthol-6-sulfonic acid. Some of the cresidine sulfonic acid may also be further acetylated. All these metabolites are likely to be excreted in the urine and very little is likely to be excreted in the bile (17).

Long-term studies in rats showed no adverse effects, except moderate growth depression at the highest level tested. However, this study was considered to be inadequate because of the poor survival and small number of animals examined terminally. Studies on reproduction and embryotoxicity including teratogenicity revealed no significant adverse effects in the two species investigated (rat, rabbit). A two-year study in dogs showed no compound-related toxic effects.

No acceptable daily intake for man (ADI) has been established for this color because of the lack of metabolic studies and the unsatisfactory nature of the sole long-term study in rat available for evaluation (18).

This color was re-evaluated subsequently when some metabolic studies using radio-labeled materials were made available. These studies demonstrated that the metabolism of this color is imilar to that of other members of the azo dye class (19).

Indicated areas for further investigation comprise life-span studies in the rat and mouse (20,21).

This color was listed among colors for which an acceptable daily intake for man (ADI) could not be established and these which are not toxicologically acceptable for use in food by the Scientific Committee for Food of the Commission of the European Communities (76).

One review on the toxicology of this compound (17) and one review on its specifications (168) are available. Analytical aspects can be found in reference 261.

ALUMINIUM (METAL)

Various aluminium salts are used in food technology as buffering, neutralizing, and firming agents. However, aluminium in the present context refers only to aluminium metal used as a silvering decoration in food for surface coloring.

Extensive data on metabolism is available on aluminium salts and aluminium metal. A number of short- and long-term studies in several species of animals are also available, as well as mutagenicity, reproduction studies, and observations in man.

An acceptable daily intake for man (ADI) was not considered to be necessary, since the use of aluminium metal as surface colorant is very limited and is not considered to represent a hazard to human health (22).

The Scientific Committee for Food of the Commission of the European Communities has listed this color among those colors for which an acceptable daily intake for man (ADI) could not be established, but which are nevertheless acceptable for use in food for external coloring and decorating of food only. Furthermore, it recommended that the general problem of the total intake of aluminium from all sources be studied in the future (77).

One review on the toxicology of this substance (23) and one on its specifications and methods of analysis (262) are available.

AMARANTH

This monoazo color was first synthesized in 1878. Large-scale production in the U.S. was first reported in 1914. In 1921, this amounted to 14,500 kg and in 1972 six U.S. companies manufactured about 440,000 kg. There are probably 18 producers of amaranth in Western Europe, with a combined total annual production of approximately 300,000 kg. The color has been approved for food use in many countries throughout the world. Known exceptions are Finland, Yugoslavia and the USSR. In the U.S., amaranth was used in the coloring of gelatin, maraschino cherries, sausage casings, frozen desserts, carbonated beverages, dry drink powders, sweets and confectionery products not containing oils and fats, bakery products and cereals, puddings, aqueous drug solutions, tablets, capsules, mouthwashes, bath salts, and hair rinses. It has been reported to have been used in at least 1,370 drug products (24).

Many toxicological studies have been carried out in several animal species. Biochemical studies in rats show that a major portion of the color is reduced at the azo-linkage, apparently by intestinal bacteria. In a previous evaluation, a no-effect level in the rat was considered to be 3,000 ppm in the diet corresponding to 150 mg/kg bw and the toxicological data were considered sufficient for recommending an ADI for man of 1.5 mg/kg bw (25).

In a subsequent evaluation, the ADI for man was adjusted to 0.75 mg/kg bw, temporarily due to the inability of making a final re-evaluation, since further relevant studies were in progress, because there were conflicting results regarding its fetus toxicity, and the difficulty in interpreting studies regarding its carcinogenic potential (26,27).

The previous difficulties with amaranth, concerning potential carcinogenicity and teratogenicity, have been subsequently evaluated in the light of new data. Several new studies on reproduction and teratogenicity were available for evaluation. These gave some conflicting results with regard to fetotoxicity, although none of them produced any evidence of teratogenic effects related to amaranth administration. Further studies to elucidate the observations generating concern over reproductive effects, have shown in retrospect, apparent adverse effects because of the unexpectedly low fetal resorption in control animals compared with non-contemporary controls. An extensive comparative study has failed to reproduce these effects in the same strain. The single positive teratogenic study suffered from an inadequate specification for the dye employed.

Of the many long-term studies carried out in mice, rats, and dogs, only two indicated a carcinogenic potential not seen in any of the other studies. The problem appears to have arisen from the use, in some of the tests, of samples of amaranth with specifications different from those established by the committee. These studies were also evaluated in another report (28) where it was similarly concluded that, because of the uncertainty about the impurity content of the amaranth employed in these two studies, the carcinogenicity of this compound could not be evaluated (29).

It was concluded that toxicological evidence indicates that this product, when it complies with the established specifications, justifies the maintenance of the temporary acceptable daily intake for man of 0.75

mg/kg bw (30).

The Scientific Committee for Food of the Commission of the European Communities, after considering many additional data on reproduction, teratology, and long-term studies, endorsed the establishment of the temporary ADI for man of 0.75 mg/kg bw and it requested the results of further long-term and reproduction studies in progress (78).

In a further evaluation, a recent collaborative teratogenicity study in three different laboratories using two strains of rats, did not reveal any adverse effect when the compound was administered at 200 mg/kg bw daily by gavage or in the drinking water. Similarly, no teratogenic response was observed when cats received dietary levels of amaranth up to 264 mg/kg bw daily. In addition to these recent studies, a long-term study in rats was available, but, due to technical inadequacies, this study was not amenable to evaluation.

It was also observed that the chemical structure of amaranth did not indicate that it would be a potential carcinogen when given orally. However, because of its potentially wide usage, it was decided that additional long-term feeding studies should be undertaken. The previously established temporary acceptable daily intake of 0.75 mg/kg bw was, thus, extended. Areas for further investigations comprise long-term studies in two animal species, one including exposure in utero and through lactation (31,32,39).

Six reviews on the toxicology of this compound (33,34,35,36,37,40) and two reviews on its specifications (38,34) are available.

ANNATTO EXTRACTS

Annatto extracts in oil are obtained by extraction of the pericarp of the fruit Bixa Orellana; their color is a red solution or suspension, and bixin (the mono methyl ester or norbixin) is the principal coloring principle. Aqueous annatto extracts are obtained by extraction of the pericarp of the same fruit by means of solutions of alkali hydroxides; their color is a red alkaline dispersion or red paste, and the principal coloring compound is the disodium or dipotassium salt of norbixin. Bixin may be obtained as orange to purple plates when crystallized from acetone. It is insoluble in water, slightly soluble in ethanol, and readily soluble in ether and oils (41,42).

These substances were evaluated in 1969, and a temporary acceptable daily intake for man of 1.25 mg/kg bw has been established, based on a demonstrated no-effect level in the rat (250 mg/kg bw/day 43,44). In 1974, these substances were re-examined and the previously allocated temporary acceptable daily intake for man was extended (45,46).

The Scientific Committee for Food of the Commission of the European Communities endorsed the temporary acceptable daily intake for man (ADI) of 1.25 mg/kg bw expressed as bixin. It requested that the results of the metabolic studies reported to be in progress, be presented for evaluation. The metabolic and other biological data must be related to the main pigment in the annatto extracts, not to another geometrical isomer (78).

No data are available on the metabolism of these materials or any of their major components. Adequate long-term tests in two animal species have been performed on a well-defined type of extract containing 0.2-2.6 percent of carotenoid expressed as bixin. Short-term tests in two other species suggest a lack of cumulative action even at levels of 15 percent carotenoid in vegetable oil, or 10 percent in water. The long-term study in the rat provides a basis for evaluation. However, information on the metabolism is lacking. The dog studies indicate that the high levels of carotenoids do not produce adverse effects (46).

Indicated areas for further research comprise metabolic studies on the major carotenoids of annatto (44,46,47). Three reviews on the toxicology of these substances (48,49,50) and three reviews on their specifications (51,52,53) are available.

ANTHOCYANINS

Anthocyanins are glycosides of 2-phenylbenzopyrylium salts, mostly hydroxy-derivatives. Anthocyanidins are the aglycones of anthocyanins (54). This class of coloring materials is characterized by a complex nature and is responsible for the red, violet, and blue pigmentation of flowers, leaves, and fruit. Hydroxylation, methylation, and the formation of glycoside linkages affect color characteristics. At least six major anthocyanin compounds (anthocyanidins) have been characterized chemically: pelargonidin, cyanidin, peonidin, delphinidin, petunidin, malvidin. They occur in nature as the 3-monoglucosides and the 3,5-diglucosides. All anthocyanins are soluble in water (55,56).

These natural colorants were not evaluated because of the lack of toxicological information and the lack of knowledge of composition, the variation in composition according to the source, and the method of preparation employed (14). Information sufficient to prepare tentative specifications was available for only one food color product; anthocyanin from grape skins (56). However, because of the lack of toxicological information, no acceptable daily intake for man (ADI) has been established.

The existing biological data concerning anthocyanins are related to their pharmacological properties, the goitrogenic effects of flavonoids, the effect on the human retina, and cytoenzymological effects. References to these studies can be found in Table III.

The Scientific Committee for Food of the Commission of the European Communities decided that anthocyanins, prepared from natural foods by physical processes, could be accepted for use as coloring matter in food without further investigation (79).

No reviews on the toxicology of these substances are available. Specifications published in reference 54 were revised (56) and published together with analytical aspects (263).

AURAMINE

This compound is manufactured industrially from dimethylaniline and formaldehyde, which react to form Michler's base (tetramethyl-diamino-diphenyl methane). This base is subsequently converted to auramine by heating it with sulfur and ammonium chloride in the presence of ammonia (57).

The free base of auramine is used to prepare solvent yellow 34, a solvent soluble yellow dye. Auramine is used as a powerful antiseptic for use in nose and ear surgery in the United Kingdom. Also, in the same country, a specially purified auramine, sold under the name of Glauramine[R], is used as an antiseptic in the treatment of gonorrhea. Auramine has been used in some countries as a food dye. It is also used as a smoke dye (57).

This color has been classified in the category of food colors found to be harmful, and which should not be used in food (58,59).

The toxicological evidence on which this decision was based is partially found in references 60 and 57.

Auramine is carcinogenic in the mouse and the rat. Given orally, it has produced liver tumors in these two species. No tumors were obtained

in the only experiment performed on the dog and rabbit. The purity of
the compound used in these experiments is not known. One epidemiological
study indicates that the open manufacture of auramine presents an occupational bladder cancer risk (61).

One review on the toxicology of this compound (62) and one on its
specifications (63) are available.

AZORUBINE

Azorubine, also called carmoisine (the former is a preferable name
since the latter can be confused with Fast Red 3, C.I. 16045) is a
monoazo compound first synthesized in 1885. In 1972, it was manufactured
in the UnitedStates by five companies and production data were included
in a group of at least 33 other acid red colors with a total production
of 642,000 kg. In Western Europe, there are probably 15 manufacturers
who produce this color, and it is believed that current production is
more than 100,000 kg per year. In Japan, one manufacturer reported production of 4,000 kg in 1973 and 2,700 kg in 1972. It is extensively
used for coloring food, cosmetics, and drugs in a number of countries
(64). Azorubine is not known to occur in nature.

Little information is available on the metabolism of this color.
It has been adequately long-term studied in the mouse. The long-term
studies in the rat recorded only tumor incidence and survival, while
many other essential observations have not been reported. A reproduction
study did not reveal any compound-related adverse effects. No-effect
level has been demonstrated in the rat at a level of 2,000 ppm in the
diet (equivalent to 100 mg/kg bw. This level has been used as a basis
for the establishment of a temporary acceptable daily intake for man at
0.5 mg/kg bw (65).

However, the Scientific Committee for Food of the Commission of the
European Communities, after considering additional information on long-
term teratogenicity studies, established a temporary acceptable daily
intake for man of 2 mg/kg bw, and requested the results of an adequate
long-term study in another species, as well as metabolic studies in
several species, and if possible, in man (66).

This color was tested for carcinogenicity in mice and rats by the
oral and subcutaneous routes. The test by the oral route in mice was
negative. The other studies could not be evaluated for carcinogenic potential because of the small numbers of animals used. No case reports or
epidemiological studies were available (67).

In a subsequent evaluation, new studies were examined. A no-effect
level of 250 mg/kg bw was demonstrated in a 90-day feeding study in rats.
Based on these new toxicological data, the previously established temporary acceptable daily intake was changed to a new temporary ADI of
1.25 mg/kg bw and the previously indicated areas for further investigation (68,69) were modified to include a long-term feeding study in rats;
a one-year feeding study in a non-rodent mammalian species; and metabolic
studies, in several species, preferably including man (39).

Four reviews on the toxicology of this compound (40,70,71,72) and
four on its specifications (73,74,75,264) are available. General analytical methods are found in reference 265.

BEET RED

This natural colorant is a red aqueous sugar-containing press juice,
a dark-red concentrate, or a reddish powder; it contains about 1 percent betanine (the major coloring principle) when in the form of a press

juice, or 4 percent betanine when in form of powder. These extracts are obtained from beets (80,81).

There is no information available on the metabolism of this naturally occurring betanine. The available long-term and reproduction studies are inadequate because only a few parameters were examined and many other essential observations have not been reported. No specific information is available on embryotoxicity including teratogenicity. This color is, however, a normal constituent of food. Although the primary criteria are the same for evaluating the safety of food colors of natural or synthetic origin, consideration must be given to the quantities of food color ingested as a result of technological use, relative to its ingestion as an ingredient of food. This and the availability of adequate chemical specifications permitted the allocation of a temporary acceptable daily intake "not specified" in the absence of a full range of toxicological investigations (83).

The Scientific Committee for Food of the Commission of the European Communities did not endorse the above decision, but felt able to accept the use of this coloring matter in food without the need for further investigations. Metabolic studies in several species and, if possible, in man, and an adequate long-term study in one acceptable species will be needed if considerable extension of the use in food of this color is contemplated (79).

In a subsequent evaluation, the increasing interest in use of this color in foods was noted. In view of the structure of the major coloring principle, betanine, a full toxicological evaluation of this compound was deemed necessary, but the previously established temporary ADI "not specified" was extended. Regarding betanine, it was noted that this coloring principle had been isolated for commercial use, however, only limited information was available on it. The previously indicated areas for further investigations (83,84) were modified to include a long-term feeding study in two animal species, a short-term feeding study in a non-rodent mammalian species, and a multigeneration feeding study including teratogenicity and metabolic studies in several species, preferably including man (39).

One review on the toxicology of these materials (85) and three reviews on their specifications (81,86,721) are available. Information is also found in reference 87.

BENZYL VIOLET 4B

This triarylmethane compound was used in the U.S. as a color additive for food, drugs, and cosmetics until 1973. Food uses were in meat inks, sweets and confections, pet foods, beverages, bakery goods, ice-cream, sherbet, dairy products, snack foods, gelatine desserts, and puddings. Pharmaceutical products in which it was used were lipsticks, rouges, hair rinses, and temporary color shampoos. It does not appear on any lists of colorants permitted for use in food in the European Economic Communities; however, some member states may use it in food until 1980. It may be used in cosmetics, including those which may be in contact with mucous membranes. In Switzerland, it is used as a dyestuff; and in Japan, it is used to dye leather, paper, and inks (88).

Biochemical and metabolic data is scarce; from these data it appears that the absorption of the dye in the gastrointestinal tract is low (23).

This color is carcinogenic in rats following its oral or subcutaneous administration. It produced mammary carcinomas and squamous-cell carcinomas of the skin after its oral administration to female rats, and local fibrosarcomas following its subcutaneous injection in male and female rats. It also increased the incidence of benign mammary tumors in female rats, following ambient exposure. No case reports or epidemiological studies are available on this compound (89). While the carcinogenic response might be due to an active impurity in the material used in the long-term studies, pending the isolation and identification of the specific carcinogenic entity in the color, this material should not be used in foods (90).

Two reviews on the toxicology of this compound (23,91) and two on its chemical specifications (92,93) are available. Information can also be found in reference 94.

BLACK 7984

This disazo compound is the tetrasodium of 6-amino-4-hydroxy-1- 7-sulfo-4- (p-sulfophenyl)azo -1-naphthyl azo -2,7-naphthalenedisulfonic acid (95). It has been classified, in the past, as a color for which the available data were inadequate for evaluation, and for which no information on long-term toxicity was available; colors with long-term tes tests for tumor formation unaccompanied by other long-term studies were considered as falling within this category (96,97,98).

The dye is poorly absorbed from the gastrointestinal tract after oral administration to rats. The data on metabolism is very scarse, however, after intravenous injection a rapid reductive splitting of the azo linkages between the two naphthalene rings occurs. One long-term study in rats produced no evidence of tumors and a two-generation reproduction study showed no gross adverse effects; however, the parameters studied in these tests are deficient (23).

The long-term studies available on this color were not considered adequate with regard to number of animals and histopathological examination. In addition, the reproduction studies lacked sufficient details to permit evaluation. No acceptable daily intake for man (ADI) could be established pending the availability of studies meeting the requirements outlined for toxicological evaluation of food colors (99).

The Scientific Committee for Food of the Commission of the European Communities endorsed the decision not to establish an ADI for this color, because of the inadequacy of the available data, and it decided that this compound is not acceptable for use in food (76).

One review on the toxicology of this compound (23) and one on its chemical specifications (100) are available.

BLUE VRS

This triphenylmethane compound is the sodium salt of 4- alpha- p-(diethylamino)phenyl -2,4-disulfobenzylidine 2,5-cyclohexadien-1-ylidene diethylammonium hydroxide, inner salt (101). Its coloring properties were first described in 1902 (102).

Some confusion exists in the classification of literature for this material, since patent blue V (C.I. 42051) has been classified under blue VRS (103).

Blue VRS was used in the past as a food dye; however, presently, it does not appear on any current lists of dyes permitted for use in food in the U.S., Japan, or the European Economic Communities. It is provisionally accepted for use in cosmetics in which it does not come into contact with mucous membranes (104).

This colorant has been classified, in the past, as a color for which the available data were inadequate for evaluation, and for which no information on long-term toxicity was available; colors with long-term tests for tumor formation, unaccompanied by other long-term studies, were considered as falling within this category (96,105). No acceptable daily intake for man (ADI) had been established.

This dye exhibits high plasma protein binding. No data on the embryotoxicity, teratogenicity, or mutagenicity are available. It is carcinogenic in rats following its subcutaneous or intramuscular injection, and produces sarcomas at the site of repeated injection. No case reports or epidemiological studies are available (106).

One review on the toxicology of this compound (103) and one on its chemical specifications (105) are available. Information can also be found in reference 107.

BRILLIANT BLACK PN

This disazo compound has been classified, in the past, as a color for which the available data were inadequate for toxicological evaluation, and for which no information on long-term toxicity was available; colors with long-term tests for tumor formation unaccompanied by other long-term studies were considered as falling within this category (96, 108). Little was known of its metabolism and only one long-term study on tumor incidence in one animal species was available. Parenteral administration of this compound did not induce any local neoplastic changes (109).

In a subsequent evaluation, it was observed that the earlier long-term studies in rats using oral administration in the diet and drinking water did not reveal carcinogenicity, but were inadequate with regard to the numbers of animals used and the parameters studied. Later long-term studies in the mouse and rat did not reveal any significant adverse effects due to administration of the compound. A no-effect level has been demonstrated in long-term studies for the rat (500 mg/kg bw/day) and a temporary ADI for man of 2.5 mg/kg bw was established (110,111).

In a further evaluation, a long-term mouse feeding study and a 90-day feeding study in pigs were considered. The mouse study revealed no significant adverse effects. In the case of the pig study, intestinal cysts were noted at the two highest feeding levels. On the basis of the additional toxicological data, the previously established ADI was extended, but it was felt that the aetiology and pathology of the cysts should be elucidated and the previously indicated areas for further investigations (110) were modified to include metabolic studies in several species, preferably including man; adequate reproduction studies including a teratogenicity study, and studies to elucidate the significance of the intestinal cysts observed in the pig study (39).

The Scientific Committee for Food of the Commission of the European Communities, after considering additional toxicological studies on this compound departed from the above decision and established an acceptable daily intake for man (ADI) of 0.75 mg/kg bw and requested the results of metabolic studies in several species and, if possible, in man; reproduction including embryotoxicity and teratogenicity studies; and full details still outstanding of studies so far reported. These results should be submitted before 1980 (78).

Four reviews on the toxicology of this compound (112,113,114,40) and four reviews on its chemical specifications (115,116,117,266) are available. General methods of analysis can be found in reference 265.

BRILLIANT BLUE FCF

This triarylmethane compound's common name, brilliant blue FCF, has been applied to both the diammonium and disodium salts. Some confusion exists in the classification of the literature for these compounds.

Although most is classified under the diammonium salt, the disodium salt is the one of primary commercial importance. The disodium salt is used in foods, and the diammonium salt appears to have had limited usage, only in drugs and cosmetics (118).

The diammonium salt is not permitted for food use in the U.S. or Japan, nor is it included in the list of colorants permitted for use in food in the European Economic Communities. Brilliant blue FCF, diammonium salt is permitted for use in the European Economic Communities in cosmetics which come into contact with mucous membranes (119).

The disodium salt is provisionally listed in the U.S. subject to certification, for use in food, drugs, and cosmetics: it occurs as a food color in beverages, sweets and confections, bakery goods, pudding powders, ice cream, sherbet, daily products, pet foods, cereals, sausages, maraschino cherries, snack foods, and meat inks. It is used to color aqueous drugs, tablets, and capsules, and its aluminum lake is used in ointments. The cosmetics in which it can occur include bath salts and hair rinses, and its aluminum lake is used in lipsticks, rouges, face powders, and talcums. In Japan, it is approved for use as a food color in all but the following foods: beans, fresh fish and shellfish, fresh vegetables, and other foods (120).

The compound was, in the past, classified in the category of colors for which the available toxicological data were not entirely sufficient to meet the requirements for establishing an acceptable daily intake for man (ADI). Extensive long-term studies were available in several animal species. At the highest level used, no pathological changes or other adverse effects were observed. Local sarcomas were produced only on repeated subcutaneous injections. However, the paucity of biochemical data made it impossible to carry out a toxicological assessment (121). Subsequently, it was again considered and the available data permitted an assessment of the toxicological potential of this color following the clarification of the significance of local sarcomas after subcutaneous injections (122).

The production of a high percentage of local sarcomas at the site of subcutaneous injection in rats has led in the past to considerable discussion and, consequently, to extensive studies on this color. The production of these sarcomas is considered to be related to the physico-chemical properties of the color and special condition of the experiment and does not constitute evidence of carcinogenicity by the oral route.

Biochemical studies have shown that the color is poorly absorbed and is almost completely excreted in the feces after parenteral administration. Extensive long-term studies in two species are available. In addition a 13-week study in rats with o-sulfobenzaldehyde, one of the components of commercial brilliant blue FCF, has been carried out. Oral feeding produced no pathological changes at the highest levels used in adequate experiments.

A no-effect level has been demonstrated in long-term studies for the rat (2500 mg/kg bw/day) and an ADI for man of 12.5 mg/kg bw was established (123,124).

The Scientific Committee for Food of the Commission of the European Communities, after considering additional long-term reproduction, and teratogenicity studies, did not endorse this decision and it established a temporary acceptable daily intake for man (ADI) of 2.5 mg/kg bw (78).

In a recent assessment of the carcinogenic potential of this compound, it has been noted that brilliant blue FCF, disodium salt, is carcinogenic in rats after its subcutaneous injection: it produced fibrosarcomas following repeated injections. It also produced an increased incidence of kidney tumors in mice after its oral administration (125).

Indicated areas for further desirable research comprise biochemical studies on metabolism using modern techniques (123).

Four reviews on the toxicology of this compound (118,126,127,128) and two reviews on its chemical specifications (129,130) are available.

BROWN FK

This disazo mixture has been classified, in the past, as a color for which the available data were inadequate for a toxicological evaluation, and for which no information on long-term toxicity was available; colors with long-term tests for tumor formation unaccompanied by other long-term studies were considered as falling within this category (96, 131).

The metabolism and toxicity of this material have been adequately studied; however, reproduction and teratogenicity studies are inadequate. The studies involving metabolites show that two major effects need to be considered; the degenerative lesions, and the deposition of a brown pigment in various organs and tissues of experimental animals. Both effects appear to be dose-related. There is good evidence that the primary metabolites, 1,2,4-triaminobenzene and 2,4,5-triaminotoluene, are cardiotoxic (23). In long-term studies in mice, this material produced hepatic nodules and tissue pigmentation. It was also shown to be mutagenic in microbial systems upon metabolic activation. The material tested contained about 50 percent impurities. Several of these impurities have been identified and some data are available on their metabolism in animals. Due to the above reasons, no acceptable daily intake for man (ADI) could be established (132).

The Scientific Committee for Food of the Commission of the European Communities, however, in an earlier assessment, established a temporary acceptable daily intake for man (ADI) of 0.05 mg/kg bw for this material, and requested further long-term study in another strain of rats, as well as reproduction and teratological studies. The Committee further recommended that in carrying out the long-term study, the nitrite level in the diet of experimental animals should be estimated as an additional parameter (133).

One review on the toxicology of this material (23) and one on its chemical specifications (131) are available. Information can also be found in reference 134.

BUTTER YELLOW

This monoazo compound was first prepared in 1876. It can be synthesized by reacting aniline with dimethylaniline, followed by the addition of sodium nitrite in a sodium hydroxide solution.

In the U.S., it was withdrawn from the approved list of food additives in 1918, six months after its addition to the list, because contact dermatitis was observed in factory workers handling it (135). It was classified as a color found to be harmful and which should not be used in food (136,137).

Since 1954, this color has been known to be a very active carcinogen in rats and a weak carcinogen in mice. In typical experiments in which the dye was fed at the level of 0.06 percent (600 ppm) in the diet, all the rats normally developed liver cancer within six months (138).

In a more recent evaluation of its carcinogenic potential, it was observed that this compound is carcinogenic in rats, producing liver tumors after its administration by several routes; and in dogs, producing bladder tumors following its oral administration. Results of oral administration studies were doubtful in mice, and negative in hamsters and guinea-pigs; but these studies were of short duration, and the adequacy of the dose levels used was not known. The compound has also been tested by subcutaneous injection in mice, and the results are suggestive of local and hepatic carcinogenicity. Treatment of newborn animals produced systemic carcinogenic effects in mice; however, the negative results obtained in rats are doubtful, since the period of observation was too short.

Skin painting with butter yellow produced epidermal tumors in rats but not in mice. An extensive dose-response study was carried out in rats; the lowest effective dose was 1 mg/rat/day and the highest noneffective dose 0.3 mg/rat/day (139).

Two reviews on the toxicology of this compound (138,140) are available.

CANTHAXANTHIN

This carotenoid was detected for the first time in an edible mushroom, the chanterelle (Cantharellus cinnabarinus). It was subsequently shown to be present in the plumage and organs of flamingos and various exotic birds, such as the scarlet ibis (Guara rubra) and the roscato spoonbill (Ajaja ajaja). It has recently been detected in various crustacea and fish (trout, salmon) (141).

Canthaxanthine is predominantly the trans-isomer and contains no less than 96 percent and no more than the equivalent of 101 percent of $C_{40}H_{52}O_2$, and appears as deep violet crystals. The articles of commerce may be solutions in oil, fat, or organic solvents; or water dispersible forms such as powders or granules that are orange to red in color (142). In an earlier evaluation of this substance, two levels of acceptable daily intake for man (ADI) were established (conditional: 12.5 mg/kg bw; unconditional: 25 mg/kg bw) based on a demonstrated no-effect level in the rat (2,500 mg/kg bw/day) (143,144). In a subsequent evaluation, and in line with provisions to abolish allocations of conditional acceptable daily intake figures (145), the acceptable daily intake for man for this substance was fixed at 25 mg/kg bw, based on the previously demonstrated no-effect level in the rat (2,500 mg/kg bw/day) (146,147).

Canthaxanthin has been adequately tested in the rat in a three-generation reproduction study and in a long-term study. It did not exhibit provitamin A activity and no adverse effects were found at the highest level tested (147).

The Scientific Committee for food of the Commission of the European Communities endorsed the ADI decision (148).

Two reviews on the toxicology of this substance (141,149) and two reviews on its specifications (142,150) are available.

CAPSANTHIN/CAPSORUBINE

These coloring principles of paprika (Capsicum annuum) are not currently manufactured products. The available information on dry paprika products used as food coloring is not sufficient to prepare specifications, nor to carry out a toxicological evaluation, owing to lack of toxicological data (151).

No toxicological reviews or specifications for these products are available.

CARAMEL COLORS

Caramel refers to a large number of ill-defined and complex products formed from various carbohydrates, by heating them with any of a wide range of acids, bases and salts, under different conditions of temperature and pressure (152).

Different grades of caramels are sometimes described as being "single strength" or "double strength," based on their tinctorial capacity. The amounts of fixed nitrogen or sulfur dioxide are higher in "double strength" caramels. It is understood that "double strength" caramels are used in amounts equal to or less than one'half the amounts of "single strength" caramels to achieve the same color effect in the final food product (153).

Generally, caramel colors contain 50 percent digestible carbohydrate, 25 percent non-digestible carbohydrate, and 25 percent of malanoidins also found in roasted coffee, broiled meats, and baked cereal products (154). Caramel colors made by the ammonia process contain traces of 4-methylimidazole and other nitrogen-containing heterocyclic compounds. The formation of these heterocyclic compounds in glucose-ammonia reactions is a function of the ratio of the reactants: The higher the molar ratio of ammonia to glucose, the greater will be the proportion of heterocyclic compounds present in the final caramel product. Other reaction conditions can also influence the proportion of heterocyclic compounds formed (153).

The 4-methylimidazole content of these caramels, together with the sulfur dioxide content and the ammoniacal nitrogen content, can generally be related to the tinctorial capacity of the product where that capacity falls within the range of 20,000-90,000 European Brewery Convention (EBC) units (155).

The production of violent hysteria and convulsions in cattle and sheep fed ammoniated sugar-containing feed supplements (nitrogen content 4-6 percent, at 6-25 percent of their rations) led to the discovery of the presence of about 20 percent of pyrazines and 10 percent of imidazoles in these ammonium-treated molasses. 4-methylimidazole has been shown to be the most likely toxic component, being a convulsant to rabbits, mice, and chicks at oral doses of 360 mg/kg bw.

The pyrazines, on the other hand, are mild depressants of the central nervous system (CNS) and weak anticonvulsants. Analysis of food grade caramel colors, however, showed that only 0.002-0.02 percent of 4-methylimidazole is present in commercial products. Commercial caramel colors of undefined origin contain 50-500 ppm 4-methylimidazole, while other examinations have shown ranges of 100-700 ppm. It has been shown that the yields of imidazole compounds increased linearly with the increment of molar ratio of ammonia to glucose (154,156).

When first examined, no decision was made concerning the safety of caramel colors produced with ammonia or ammonium salts process, because of the concern over the toxicity of 4-methylimidazole (157). When subsequently evaluated, an acceptable daily intake for man (ADI) "not specified"* was allocated to caramel colors produced by processes other than

---

*The statement "ADI not specified" means that, on the basis of the available data (toxicologial, biochemical, and other), the total daily intake of the substance, arising from its use or uses at the levels necessary to achieve the desired effect and from its acceptable background in food, does not, in the opinion of the committee (Joint FAO/WEO Expert Committee on Food Additives), represent a hazard to health. For this reason, and for the reasons stated in the individual evaluation, the establishment of an acceptable daily intake for man (ADI in mg/kg bw is not deemed necessar

those utilizing ammonia, and a temporary ADI of 100 mg/kg bw was allocated to caramel colors produced by the ammonia process; this ADI was based on a demonstrated no-effect level in rats (10,000 mg/kg bw/day) (158,159).

In a further examination of these products, the temporary ADI was extended for an additional period of time; however, it has been pointed out that the figure of 100 mg/kg bw should be related to a product having a color intensity of 20,000 EBC (European Brewery Convention) units and containing no more than 200 mg/kg (200 ppm) of 4-methylimidazole (160,161). A large number of caramel color has been tested in short-term studies and one variety has been tested in dogs. The acute and short-term studies considered reveal that high levels of intake have no adverse effects on the CNS (central nervous system).

Therefore, the acute neurological effects produced by high doses of 4-methylimidazole would not appear to be of major concern hen caramel colors containing small amounts of this contaminant are used in food. The analytical evidence suggests the presence of 4-methylimidazole in the range of 50-700 ppm in caramel colors, depending upon the process of manufacture; 200 ppm is taken as an average low value for 4-methylimidazole content. Since the effects of chronic ingestion of 4-methyl are unknown, the above-mentioned long-term studies, as well as more adequate reproduction, embryotoxicity including teratology studies, have been recommended on caramel colors produced by the ammonia-ammonium sulfate process (161).

In a subsequent evaluation, the existing chemical specifications for caramel colors produced by the ammonia process were found to be ambiguous, since they appeared to cover colors manufactured by the ammonia-sulfite process as well. More accurate definition of the products permitted separate specifications to be established for caramel colors produced by the ammonia process and those produced by the ammonia-sulfite process.

Since the last evaluation of these substances, much additional information has become available. This information shows that the two types of caramel colors differ in their toxicity. The principal toxic effect of ammoniated caramel appears to be depression of circulating lymphocytes and leukocytes. Feeding studies with both types of caramels also have demonstrated pigment deposition in mesenteric lymph nodes. However, this latter effect was considered to be a physiological response. In addition, teratogenicity studies with these substances have not demonstrated any adverse effect.

In short-term studies with rats fed ammoniated caramel, a no-effect level for lymphocyte depression was not demonstrated. The lowest level fed was 0.5 percent of the diet. A similar effect was noted in long-term rat studies at 3 percent of the diet. Lower levels have not been adequately tested in long-term studies. Since a no-effect level could not be demonstrated, the temporary ADI for non-sulfited ammoniated caramel was revoked.

With regard to ammoniated sulfited caramels, toxicological evaluation is complicated by conflicting results on the effects of these substances on circulating lymphocytes and leukocytes. Although 4-methylimidazole is no longer considered to be a concern, and the introduction of chemical specifications has limited its concentration, it has been decided to maintain the limit for this substance in specifications to indicate good manufacturing practices. An ADI for man of 100 mg/kg bw was retained for the sulfited ammoniated caramels. This ADI is temporary, until data from an adequate chronic study are reviewed (162).

The Scientific Committee for Food of the Commission of the European Communities endorsed the decision of allocating separate ADI to caramels prepared by different processes: an ADI without a specified upper limit to caramel color made by other than the ammonia process, and a temporary ADI of 100 mg/kg bw to caramel color prepared by ammonia or ammonium sulfite process (163). No distinction has been made between the two processes; ammonia or ammonium sulfite.

Indicated areas for further investigation comprise adequate carcinogenicity/teratogenicity studies for sulfited ammoniated caram ls, with particular attention to bone marrow and immune competence (162).

Three reviews on the toxicology of these substances (154,164,165) and two on their specifications (166,167) are available. Separate specifications for caramel color; plain, ammonia process, and ammonia-sulfite process, as well as analytical methods and methods for determination of color intensity can be found in reference 267.

CARBON BLACKS

Carbon blacks are obtained by the heating of different types of organic material. They are fine, bulky, black powders; insoluble in water; and may contain a considerable amount of inorganic ash, particularly those produced from charcoal (169).

Two types of source materials that have been used as food coloring agents can be used to manufacture carbon blacks. Carbon blacks made from vegetable materials, such as peat, differ considerably from products based on hydrocarbons such as natural gas, with respect to ash content and other impurities. The content of polynuclear aromatic hydrocarbons (PNAs) depends on the nature of the source material and the carbonizing conditions, especially the temperature, and the time at high temperature. Analytical methods applied in the past have not resolved the question of how strongly and irreversibly PNAs are absorbed in carbon black. Given the increases in sensitivity of some of the methods under study, PNAs will be detected in some extracts of carbon black. Until the levels that can be extracted are known, no limits for PNAs can be indicated (170).

Toxicological tests which have been carried out are inadequate to permit an evaluation of carbon blacks as food colorants. These studies are referred to in Table III.

The Scientific Committee for Food of the Commission of the European Communities listed carbon blacks and activated vegetable carbon with colors for which an ADI could not be established, but which are nevertheless acceptable for external and/or mass coloring of sugar confectionery (171).

In a subsequent evaluation, the Committee observed that the only product that complied with its earlier recommendations on limits for polycyclic aromatic hydrocarbons was, in fact, E153. The Committee has also been informed that there was an application of this coloring matter in tinting several foodstuffs. The quantities used are not large. In view of its use as a traditional therapeutic agent, the Committee was therefore able to recommend the maintenance of the substance in the directive for food use in general, despite the absence of extensive animal toxicological data (724).

No reviews on the toxicology of these substances, and only one on its specifications (169) are available.

BETA-APO-8'-CAROTENAL

This food colorant is predominantly the trans-isomer and contains no less than 96 percent and no more than the equivalent of 101 percent of $C_{30}H_{40}O$, and it appears as deep violet crystals with metallic luster.

The articles of commerce may be solutions in oil, fat, or organic solvents; or water dispersible forms such as powders or granules that are
orange to red in color (172). This su-stance is found in abundance in
the vegetable kingdom, e.g. in the pulp and skin of citrus fruits and
in various fooder plants (173).

In a previous evaluation, a two-level acceptable daily intake for
man (ADI) was allocated to beta-apo-8'-carotenal as a food colorant
(conditional: 5 mg/kg bw; unconditional: 2.5 mg/kg bw) based on a
demonstrated no-effect level for beta-carotene in the rat (50 mg/kg bw/
day), satisfactory biochemical information and its activity as provitamin A (174,175).

In a subsequent evaluation, in line with provisions to abolish
allocations of conditional ADI figures (176), the acceptable daily intake for man was fixed at 5 mg/kg bw. This figure represents the result
of a group evaluation of several substances chemically and toxicologically related (176), since the ADI figure refers to the sum of beta-apo-
8'-carotenal, beta-carotene, and the methyl and ethyl esters of beta-
apo-8'-carotenic acid (177,178,179).

Beta-apo-8'-carotenal has been adequately tested in rats. The use
of this substance is unlikely to result in an increased level of vitamin A, although the conversion rate for man is not known. Like beta-
carotene, this substance is poorly absorbed from the gastrointestinal
tract when present in large amounts (179).

The Scientific Committee for Food of the Commission of the European
Communities endorsed the figure of acceptable daily intake for man allocated to this substance (148).

Two reviews on the toxicology of this substance (173,180) and two
reviews on its specifications (181,182) are available. Analytical aspects can be found in reference 183.

CAROTENES (NATURAL)

Carotenes extracted from natural sources are colored, highly un-
saturated hydrocarbons at all-trans configuration. They occur in nature
in isomeric forms which differ in the position of the double bond in
the ionone rings, or have only one ionone ring (184). In plants, they
usually occur together with chlorophyll. The most important pigments
are alpha, beta, and gamma carotene. These three substances all have
provitamin A activity, beta- arotene being converted in vivo into two
molecules of vitamin A. The alpha and gamma isomers are capable of producing only one molecule of vitamin A per molecule of the pigment. The
most important sources of alpha-carotene are: red palm oil, green chest-
nut leaves, mountain ash berries; beta-carotene: alfalfa, carrots,
green leaves, and butter; gamma-carotene: leaves of lily of the valley,
Gonocarium pyriforme (185).

A toxicological assessment of these substances was not possible on
the data available, and because further information was required on the
chemical specifications for carotenes derived from natural sources, no
acceptable daily intake for man was allocated to these substances (178).

No reviews on the toxicology of these substances and only one on
their specifications (184) are available. Analytical aspects can be
found in reference 186.

CAROTENE, BETA-(SYNTHETIC)

Synthetic beta-carotene is predominantly the trans-isomer and contains no less than 96 percent and no more than the equivalent of 101

percent of beta-carotene ($C_{40}H_{56}$). It appears as red crystals or crystalline powder. The articles of commerce may be solutions in oils, fat, or organic solvents; or water dispersible forms such as powders or granules (187).

In a previous evaluation, a two-level acceptable daily intake for man (ADI) was established for beta-carotene (conditional: 5.0 mg/kg bw; unconditional: 2.5 mg/kg bw) based ona demonstrated no-effect level in the rat (50 mg/kg bw/day), satisfactory biochemical information, and its activity as provitamin A (188,189).

In a subsequent re-evaluation, and in line with provisions to abolish allo ations of conditional acceptable daily intake figures (176), the acceptable daily intake for man (ADI) was fixed at 5 mg/kg bw. This figure represents the result of group evaluation of several substances chemically and toxicologically related (176), since the acceptable daily intake refers to the sum of beta-apo-8'-carotenal, beta-carotene, and beta-apo-8'-carotenoic acid (ethyl and methyl esters) (177,178,190).

Beta-carotene is a normal constituent of the human diet and is commonly ingested over the entire life span of man. Its biological importance rests on the provitamin A function. Concerning the known clinical syndrome of hypervitaminosis A in man, evidence from human experience indicates that in very exceptional circumstances, excessive dietary intakes can occur. Such cases have been reported in the literature, but do not relate to food additive use of this color. Despite poor a sorption from the gastrointestinal tract, cases of human hypervitaminosis have occurred. The results of short-term toxicity studies in rats and dogs have shown that over a wide range of doses, toxic effects have not been produced. Similarly, multigeneration tests in rats, using levels up to 1,000 ppm have not revealed any adverse effects.

In light of the above comments, it appears justifiable to apply a smaller safety factor to the no-effect level established in long-term studies in the rat (191).

The Scientific Committee for Food of the Commission of the European Communities endorsed the figure of acceptable daily intake for man allocated to this substance (148).

Two reviews on the toxicology of this compound (192,193) and three reviews on its specifications (194,195,196) are available. Analytical aspects can be found in reference 197.

CAROTENOIC ACID (BETA-APO-8'-) (ETHYL AND METHYL ESTERS)

These compounds are predominantly the _trans_-isomers and contain no less than 96 percent and no more than the equivalent of 101 percent of $C_{31}H_{42}C_2$ or $C_{32}H_{44}O_2$, respectively. They appear as red crystals. The article of commerce may be solutions in oil, fat, or organic solvents; or water-dispersible forms such as powders or granules that are yellow to orange in color (198).

In a previous evaluation, a two-level acceptable daily intake for man was established (conditional: 5.0 mg/kg bw; unconditional: 2.5 mg/kg bw) based on a demonstrated no-effect level for beta-carotene in the rat (50 mg/kg bw/day), satisfactory biochemical information, and its activity as provitamin A (189,199).

In a subsequent re-evaluation, and in line with provisions to abolish allocations of conditional acceptable daily intake figures, (176) the acceptable daily intake for man for these substances was fixed at 5 mg/kg bw. This figure represents the results of group evaluation of several substances chemically and toxicologically related (176), since the acceptable daily intake refers to the sum of beta-apo-8'-carotenal, beta-carotene, and beta-apo-8'-carotenoic acid (ethyl and methyl esters) (177,178,200).

Although the toxicological information on each individual ester is incomplete, long-term studies have been reported in rats. The use of these substances is unlikely to result in an increased level of Vitamin A, although the conversion rate for man is not known. Like beta-carotene, these substances are poorly absorbed from the gastrointestinal tract, especially when present in large amounts. They can, therefore, be evaluated on the same basis as beta-carotene (201).

The Scientific Committee for Food of the Commission of the European Communities endorsed the figure of acceptable daily intake for man (ADI) allocated to this substance (148).

Two reviews on the toxicology of these compounds (200,202) and two reviews on their specifications (198,203) are available. Analytical aspects can be found in reference 204.

CARTHAMUS

Carthamus, the safflower (Carthamus tinctorius), is native of the East Indies, but is cultivated in Egypt and to some extent in Southern Europe. The coloring principle, carthamin ($C_{14}H_{14}O_7$) is obtained from the flowers. This natural food colorant appears on the permitted lists in several countries (205).

Scarce toxicological studies have been performed only on one type of carthamus, the commercial product Tanacolor-Y This product is presumed to be absorbed through the intestinal tract, as indicated by the yellow discoloration of many body tissues. It is thought that the liver plays a major role in the excretion of this color. Following a six-month period of oral administration to rats, the liver became extremely yellow; this was attributed to the "acceleration of the liver function to eliminate the substance."

The available data on acute toxicity indicate that female mice are more sensitive than male mice when the dye is administered intraperitoneally. Limited short-term feeding studies on rats are available. References to these studies are found in Table III.

Since data were lacking on long-term studies, reproduction/teratology and metabolism, no acceptable daily intake for man (ADI) was allocated to this product (206).

One review on the toxicology of this product (23) and tentative specifications for carthamus yellow and carthamus red together with analytical methods (268) are available.

CHLOROPHYLLS

Chlorophyll is the green pigment of plants. The sources generally used for producing the food color are alfalfa, lucerne, clover, and spinach. The product is a mixture of three parts of chlorophyll "a" and one part of chlorophyll "b" and enzymatic degradation products. Chemically, it can be considered to be the ester of chlorophyllin with phytol. By the action of the enzyme chlorophyllase, phytol is split off. Chlorophyll "a" crystallizes in green hexagonal plates, and chlorophyll "b" in dark-green needles. The commercial product is an intensely dark-green, aqueous, ethanolic, or oily solution of chlorophyll degradation products. It is soluble in ethanol, ether, chloroform, and benzene; insoluble in water (207).

Soluble chlorophyll has a low toxicity. Although chlorophyll has been ingested by man in his food since the dawn of history, in recent years, phytol intolerance, due to a rare inborn metabolism, has been described as the clinical syndrome of Refsum's disease. Knowledge about the use of chlorophyll as a food color may, therefore, be important to clinicians. To chlorophyll as a food additive has been allocated an acceptable daily intake for man (ADI) "not specified"* (208,209). However, in a subsequent evaluation, it was observed that chlorophyll per se in the food industry appears to have no major commercial use, mainly because of its instability. It was therefore decided that the non-use should be confirmed and subsequently the existing specification, and supposedly the ADI, revoked (217).

The Scientific Committee for Food of the Commission of the European Communities has listed chlorophyll among the colors for which an ADI could not be established, but which are nevertheless acceptable for use in food generally (79).

One review on the toxicology of this compound (209) and two reviews on specifications (210-211) are available. Further information can be found in reference 212. Information on analytical aspects of identification tests can be found in reference 213.

CHLOROPHYLL COPPER COMPLEX

This complex is obtained from chlorophyll, by partial replacement of magnesium by copper. It is available as blue-green powders, pastes, or viscous liquids, having a slight amine-like odor (214).

The copper in this complex is firmly bound. Although increased plasma levels of copper have been reported, there is no significant tissue storage, nor is there any evidence of destruction of ascorbic acid. Chlorophyll copper complex has higher toxicity when given parenterally, but this has no toxicological significance if this color is used orally. No significant chronic effects were seen in the long-term tests in rats. Changes in the copper levels in plasma may be of importance for people suffering from Wilson's disease (215).

In a previous evaluation, an acceptable daily intake for man (ADI) of 15 mg/kg bw was allocated to this complex on the basis of a no-effect level demonstrated in the rat (1,500 mg/kg bw/day)(216).

In a subsequent evaluation, since it has been reported that there was no major commercial use of chlorophyl per se in the food industry, mainly because of its instability, it was decided that the non-use should be confirmed and subsequently the existing specification, and, supposedly the ADI revoked (217). Consequently, the decision on the chlorophyll copper complex appears to have been suspended until the reports on its non-use will be confirmed (218).

The Scientific Committee for Food of the Commission of the European Communities has endorsed on ADI of 15 mg/kg bw as the sum of both chlorophyll copper complex and chlorophyllin copper complex (219).

One review on the toxicology of this complex (220) and three reviews on its specifications (221,222,223) are available. New revised tentative specifications were announced in reference 217. Analytical aspects can also be found in references 222, 223.

CHLOROPHYLLIN COPPER COMPLEX

Chlorophyllin copper complex salts (sodium or potassium) are obtained from chlorophyll by partial replacement of magnesium by copper

---

*See footnote on page 26.

and by replacing methyl and phytil ester groups with alkali. These salts usually contain between four and six percent total copper; they are available as blue-black powders, having a slight amine-like odor (224).

Any toxic effects of water soluble chlorophyllin copper complexes, are, in part, due to the free ionizable copper present in the salts. The copper, however, is firmly bound. Although increased plasma levels of copper have been reported, there is no significant tissue storage, nor is there any evidence of destruction of ascrobic acid. No significant chronic effects were seen in the long-term tests in rats (225,226).

A temporary acceptable daily intake for this complex of 15 mg/kg bw was allocated, since chemical specifications were tentative (227, 228,229). In a subsequent evaluation, chemical specifications were revised and finalized, and the ADI was more permanently established (230). The acceptable daily intake for man was based on a no-effect level demonstrated in the rat (1,500 mg/kg bw/day) (216).

The Scientific Committee for Food of the Commission of the European Communities has endorsed an ADI for man of 15 mg/kg bw as the sum of both chlorophyll copper complex and chlorophyllin copper complex (219).

Two reviews on the toxicology of this complex (231,232), and three on its specifications (233,234,235) are available. New revised specifications were announced (230) and published in reference 269. However, they were not finalized due to the absence of more precise information on the commercial products available and, in particular, the level of copper in the complex (39). Analytical aspects on identification tests can be found in references 234, 235, and 270.

CHOCOLATE BROWN FB

This food colorant is known to be a complex mixture of dyes. The toxicological data available comprise information on acute toxicity, short-term studies in pigs and rats, and long-term studies in mice and rats. However, it was not possible to relate this toxicological information to a substance with defined chemical specifications and, therefore, no evaluation was carried out on this substance (236). References to the above mentioned studies can be found in Table III.

The Scientific Committee for Food of the Commission of the European Communities noted that chocolate brown FB had no clearly defined composition and, therefore, it was not possible to relate the available biological data to an identifiable material used in food. The committee expressed the opinion that this color was not acceptable for use in food (76).

One review on the toxicology of this mixture is available (23). No specifications have been prepared, since it appears that this product is no longer manufactured as a food color additive (236). Other information can also be found in reference 237.

CHOCOLATE BROWN HT

This disazo compound has been classified, in the past, as a color for which the available data were inadequate for a toxicological assessment, and for which no information on long-term toxicity was available; colors with long-term tests for tumor formation unaccompanied by other long-term studies were considered as falling within this category (238).

Satisfactory carcinogenicity/toxicity studies on two rodent species are presently available, as well as a short-term study on a non-rodent species. However, data are lacking on reproduction and metabolism. Based on a no-effect level demonstrated in the mouse (500 mg/kg bw/day), a temporary ADI for man of 0.25 mg/kg bw was established (239).

Indicated areas for further investigation comprise multigeneration reproduction/teratology studies, as well as metabolism studies in several animal species, preferably including man (239).

The Scientific Committee for Food of the Commission of the European Communities, however, at an earlier assessment, established a temporary ADI for man of 2.5 mg/kg bw and requested that further work be done on this food colorant. Furthermore, this compound was the subject of a supplementary opinion of this group (240).

One review on the toxicology of this compound (23) and on its specifications (241,271) are available. Some information is also found in reference 242. Information on analytical aspects for identification and purity tests is found in references 243, 244, and 272.

CHRYSOIDINE

This monoazo compound can be synthesized by coupling diazotized aniline with meta-phenylenediamine, but it is not known whether this is a method used for commercial production. It appeared on lists of approved food colors in several countries (245).

It has been classified as a color found to be harmful and which should not be used in food (246,247).

The toxicological evidence on which this decision was based is partially found in references 3 and 57. Reference to pertinent studies can be found in Table III.

Chrysoidine is carcinogenic in mice following its oral administration, producing liver-cell tumors, leukemia, and reticulum-cell sarcomas (248).

One review on the toxicology of this substance (249) is available. Other information can be found in reference 250.

CHRYSOINE S

This monoazo water-soluble compound was classified as a food color for which the available data are inadequate for evaluation, and for which virtually no information on long-term toxicity is available; colors with long-term studies for tumor formation, unaccompanied by other long-term studies, were considered as falling within this category (247,251,252). In addition, it appears that no commercial sources are available for this substance as a food colorant (252).

The Scientific Committee for Food of the Commission of the European Communities endorsed the decision of not establishing an ADI for man because of the inadequacy of the available data. Furthermore, it expressed the opinion that this color is not acceptable for use in food (253).

Two reviews on the toxicology of this compound (23,254) and two on its specifications (251,255) are available. Analytical aspects on tests for identification can be found in reference 256. Other information can be found in reference 257.

CHRYSOINE SGX "SPECIALLY PURE"

This monoazo compound was classified as a food color for which the available data are inadequate for evaluation, and for which virtually no information on long-term toxicity is available; colors with long-term studies for tumor formation, unaccompanied by other long-term studies, were considered as falling within this category (246,247). The available toxicological data are referenced in Table III.

No reviews on the toxicology or specifications are available. Some information can be found in reference 258.

CITRANAXANTHIN

This carotenoid, which is synthesized by the aldol condensation of beta-apo-8'-carotenal with acetone, has been used as food additive for pigmentation of egg yolks and broilers, and it has been proposed for use as a food colorant and as a dye for cosmetic use. Citranaxanthin as a food additive is available in dry powder form, which consists of coated beadlets varying in color from orange, red to reddish-brown (273).

This compound has provitamin A activity in poultry. This property was tested in chicken liver storage tests (259).

Short-term studies on the toxicity of this compound are available (260). It has been reported that other toxicological studies are available as unpublished proprietary documents (15).

No acceptable daily intake for man has been established for this compound. There are no reviews available on the toxicology of this compound. Tentative specifications and methods of analysis can be found in reference 273.

The Scientific Committee for Food of the Commission of the European Communities, on the basis of available data, established an ADI of 0.4 mg/kg bw. In view of the metabolic transformation of citranaxanthin to vitamin A, this ADI should be included in the ADI of 5 mg/kg bw for all carotenoids with provitamin A activity established for beta-carotene, beta-apo-8'-carotenal, and the methyl and ethyl esters of beta-apo-8'-carotenoic acid.

No clear evidence exists for the natural occurrence of this carotenoid color. The available metabolic information points to conversion into vitamin A of the greater part of absorbed citranaxanthin, the remainder being deposited in various tissues, including the egg yolk of birds.

The long-term study in rats which has recently been completed (using a protocol established three or four years ago) revealed no adverse findings at all intake levels tested, the highest being 86 mg/kg bw citranaxanthin. The available six-month dog study and three-generation reproduction study in rats showed no evidence of adverse effects on the parameters studies, including reproduction and teratogenicity.

Taking into account the ADI and the small amounts of the color that would be used, no objection was expressed on toxicological grounds to the use of this color as an additive to poultry feed. However, the fact was emphasized that neither the nutritional quality of a chicken, nor that of an egg, can be judged on the basis of its color. Furthermore, no considerations were given to the implications of the practice of coloring egg yolks by adding citranaxanthin to poultry feed, except in terms of safety to the consumer (722).

CITRUS RED 2

This monoazo compound was first prepared in 1940. It is probably still being manufactured by two U.S. companies, but is not believed to be produced commercially in Western Europe or Japan. In the U.S., this color is permitted only for coloring the skins of oranges that are not intended or used for processing, at a level not exceeding 2 ppm on the basis of the weight of the whole fruit (274).

Information is available on the metabolism of this compound and several long-term studies have been performed. Two long-term studies in mice and rats gave discrepant findings with regard to bladder pathology with closely related dosage levels. Bladder papillary carcinomas were produced, but the presence of bladder stones made it difficult to judge whether the color itself possessed weak carcinogenic activity. On the other hand, there is evidence of metabolic conversion of a 1-amino-2-naphthylsulfate belonging to the group of substances known to induce bladder tumors when implanted in paraffin wax pellets.

The induction of remote malignant tumors in female mice is noteworthy. The many unexplained findings observed require further study in other strains of animals in order to confirm or refute them, and to explain the difference between oral and parenteral effects. On the basis of this evidence, the toxicological data available were judged inadequate to allow the determination of a safe level and it was recommended that this compound should not be used as a food color (275,276).

The carcinogenic potential of this color has been more recently examined, and it was concluded that it is carcinogenic in mice and rats. Following its oral administration, it produced hyperplasia and tumors of the bladder. Given subcutaneously, it produced adenocarcinomas of the lung and lymphosarcomas in female mice. Its administration in mice by bladder implantation produced carcinomas in that organ (277).

Three reviews on the toxicology of this compound (277,278,279) and one on its specifications (280) are available. Analytical aspects can be found in reference 277.

COCHINEAL, CARMINE, CARMINIC ACID

Cochineal is a red dyestuff prepared from the dried bodies of the female insect Coccus cacti (Dactylopius coccus Costa Fam. Coccidae), which are ground, and contain eggs and larvae. The insect grows on various species of the cactus Nopalea coccinellifera (Fam. Cactacea) in the Canary Islands, and Central and South America. Carminic acid, the coloring principle, is a dark reddish-brown or bright-red powder derived from the glycosidal coloring matter of cochineal, which may be as low as 10 percent. Its alkali salts and alumina lake are soluble in water and ethanolic solvents. Carmine is the aluminum or aluminum-calcium lake of carminic acid. Cochineal extract, but not carminic acid per se, is known to be used as a food color. Sufficient information is available to prepare chemical specifications for aluminum and aluminum-calcium lakes of carminic acid, but not for other types of products, including the alkali salts of carminic acid. Further information is required on the food color uses of cochineal; residual methanol; protein, and carminic acid contents of commercial cochineal extract; as well as methods of production; levels of use; and composition of the extract, including impurities such as the alkali salts of carminic acid (281,282,283).

These natural colorants were not evaluated because of the lack of toxicological information, the lack of knowledge of composition, and the variation in composition according to the source and the method of preparation employed (14).

The only adequate toxicity studies available are a short-term study in rats and teratogenicity studies in rats (carmine) and mice (lithium and sodium carmine). Due to the lack of other toxicity data, no evaluation was attempted and no acceptable daily intake (ADI) for man was established (283,284).

The Scientific Committee for Food of the Commission of the European Communities listed these products among the colors for which an ADI could not be established, but which are nevertheless acceptable for use in some alcoholic beverages on a temporary basis (285).

Two reviews on the toxicology of these products (23,286) and two reviews on their specifications (287,288) are available. Analytical aspects can be found in reference 289. Other aspects can be found in reference 290.

CONGO RED

This disazo compound has been classified as a food color for which the available toxicological data were inadequate for evaluation, and for which virtually no information on long-term toxicity was available (291). The toxicological evidence on which this decision was based has not been published in the form of a monograph; however, it can be found in an unpublished document (292).

Studies on intravenous LD_{50} in several species are available. The color was studied for teratogenic activity in female rats which were given a single intraperitoneal injection of a 2 percent aqueous solution of the color on the 80th day of pregnancy. Dosages used were 14, 20, 40 mg/100 g maternal body-weight. The dose of 40 mg was lethal: all pregnant rats died within five days after injection; 20 mg was found to be teratogenic, 15.4 percent of the survivors were malformed. The malformations produced were hydrocephalus, hydronephrosis, and ocular defects.

A dose of 250 mg/kg bw of the color was given intravenously in solutions of different pH to groups of 10 mice. The number of deaths recorded at 24 hours were: five at pH 7.25; six at pH 6.51; two at pH 5.95; and none at pH 4.50.

A dog was given 0.25 g of the color in water five times in 10 days by subcutaneous injection. In an observation period of one month, no tumors were observed.

A dose of 25-50 mg of the color was given daily by intravenous administration to pigeons for four days and to rabbits for 7-14 days. No adverse effect was observed. References to these studies can be found in Table III.

No reviews on this compound are available. Some information is found in reference 293.

EOSIN, EOSIN DISODIUM SALT

These xanthene dyes are commercially available as eosin and eosin disodium salt. Eosin is used as an intermediate in the production of eosin disodium salt and as a dye in cosmetics, such as lipsticks, rouges and face powders, and talcums. It is also used as an absorption indicator in the titration of bromide or iodine ions with silver nitrate. Eosin disodium salt is used as a dye or as an intermediate in the production of red lakes and toners used in printing. It is used as a dye for fibers such as wool, nylon, and silk; paper; inks; colored pencils; wool stains; aqueous drug solutions and apsules; soaps; lipsticks and nail polishes; and also as a biological stain (294). Their use as food colorants is not clearly established (295,296).

Eosin has been classified as a food color for which the available toxicological data were inadequate for evaluation, and for which virtually no information on long-term toxicity was available (295). The evidence on which this decision was based has not been published in the form of a monograph; however, it can be found in an unpublished document (297). References to studies reported in this document can be found in Table III.

Subsequently, eosin and its disodium salt have been examined for their carcinogenic potential. It was observed that eosin has been tested only in rats by oral and subcutaneous administration, and eosin disodium salt has been administered to rats by subcutaneous injection. The data were insufficient for an evaluation of carcinogenicity of these compounds to be made (298).

One review on the toxicology of these compounds (294) and one on the specifications of eosin and analytical aspects (295) are available. Some information may also be found in reference 296.

ERYTHROSINE

This xanthene color was classified in a category of colors for which the available toxicological data were not sufficient to meet the requirements for the establishment of an acceptable daily intake for man (299,300).

In a subsequent evaluation, a temporary ADI for man of 1.25 mg/kg was allocated to this color based on a demonstrated no-effect level in the rat (250 mg/kg bw) (301,302).

At the time of the evaluation, long-term studies in two animal species were found adequate, and it was observed that most of the color was excreted in the feces and some of the absorbed color was excreted via the bile. Elevation of protein-bound iodine levels has been observed, although no toxicological significance in relation to thyroid activity was attributed to this observed effect. Conversion to fluorescein, a nephotoxic compound, was considered possible and it was warned that this conversion should be avoided. Studies on the metabolism in several animal species and, preferably in man, as well as studies to elucidate the mechanism underlying the effect of this color on plasma-bound iodine levels were deemed necessary (302).

In a further evaluation, an ADI for man of 2.5 mg/kg bw was established, based on the same no-effect level in the rat previously demonstrated (250 mg/kg bw/day), since the toxicological evidence from the latest available information permitted the use of a smaller safety factor (303,304).

Indicated areas for further desirable investigation comprise metabolic studies, preferably including man, and studies on the mechanism underlying the effect on plasma-bound iodine (304).

The Scientific Committee for Food of the Commission of the European Communities endorsed an ADI of 2.5 mg/kg bw and considered this color as a compound for which an ADI could be established, and which is, therefore, acceptable toxicologically for use in food within the ADIs limit. Furthermore, the need to include in the specification a limit of 0.1 percent for the common impurity fluorescein was emphasized (148).

Three reviews on the toxicology of this compound (305,306,307) and four on its specifications (308,309,310,311) are available. Analytical aspects are found in references 312,313, and 314. Other information is found in reference 315.

FAST GREEN FCF

This triarylmethane color was classified in the category of colors for which the available toxicological data were not sufficient to meet the requirements for the establishment of an acceptable daily intake for man (316,317).

It is used in several countries in many food commodities; as a dye in pharmaceutical capsules, and as a histological stain in a specific test for DNA. It is not permitted for use in foods in the European Economic Communities; however, it may be used in cosmetics which come into contact with mucous membranes. It has been specifically approved for use in tinned apple sauce and tinned pears at a maximum level of 200 mg/kg, singly or in combination with other colors by the Codex Alimentarius Commission (318).

In a subsequent evaluation, it was observed that the production of a high percentage of local sarcomas at the site of subcutaneous injections in rats has in the past led to considerable discussion and, consequently, to extensive studies of this color. The production of these sarcomas was considered to be related to the physico-chemical properties of the color and the special conditions of the experiment, and does not constitute evidence of carcinogenicity when ingested orally. Biochemical studies have shown that the color is poorly absorbed and is almost completely excreted in the feces after parenteral administration. Extensive long-term studies in two animal species are available. However, biochemical studies on the metabolism using modern techniques were deemed desirable. The no-effect level demonstrated in a long-term study in the rat (2500 mg/kg bw) served as a basis for establishing an ADI for man of 12.5 mg/kg bw (319,320).

In a subsequent evaluation of the carcinogenic potential of this compound, it was observed that this color has been tested in mice and rats by oral administration, and in rats by subcutaneous injection. It was found to produce sarcomas in the rat at the site of repeated subcutaneous injections (321).

Three reviews on the toxicology of this compound (322,323,324) and two reviews on its specifications (325,326) are available. Analytical aspects are found in reference 322, and 327. Other information is found in reference 328.

FAST RED E

This monoazo compound has been classified in the category of colorants for which the available toxicological data were inadequate for evaluation, and for which virtually no information on long-term toxicity was available (329,330). The toxicological evidence on which this decision was based has not been published in the form of a monograph; however, it can be partially found in reference 331 and in an unpublished document (332).

At a concentration of 200 to 400 mg/liter, this compound inhibited the action of pepsin, but had no effect on lipase action. The rat intraperitoneal LD_{50} is in the range of 2.0 g/kg bw and the intravenous LD_{50} is in the range of 1.0-2.5 g/kg bw. Ten rats were injected subcutaneously with 0.5 ml of a 1 percent solution twice weekly for one year. The test animals were then maintained for a further 374 days. One animal developed a spindle-cell sarcoma (axillary tumor). Ten rats were administered a 0.5 percent solution of Fast Red E daily at a dose level equivalent to 0.55 g/kg bw for 454 days (equivalent to 50 g) of dye during the test period. No tumors were observed. Ten rats were fed a diet with 0.2 percent of the color. The daily intake was 0.1 percent g/kg bw until a total of 10.7 g per animal had been ingested. The rats were kept under observation for the extent of their lifetimes. No tumors were observed.

In the study, 162 male and female mice, 50 to 100 days of age, of mixed strain (derived from the mixed breeding of five different strains of mice) were maintained on diets containing the dye at dose equivalent to 1 mg/animal/day for a period of two years. An equal number of mice as negative controls, and also positive control groups with either o-aminoazotoluene or dimethylamino-azobenzene were included in the study. In the positive control group, tumors were observed at seven months. Sacrifice of test animals and controls at either 16 months or two years showed that the incidence of tumors in mice receiving the dye was not significantly greater than in negative controls. A group of ten rats was maintained on a diet containing 0.2 percent of the dye for 417 days (equivalent to a total intake of 10.7 g/rat). The rats were then maintained for a further 479 days. No tumors were observed.

Fast Red E was not mutagenic to E. coli at a concentration of 0.5 percent and it did not show sensitization activity in studies with guinea-pigs. The test for Heinz bodies was negative in four cats dosed with a 5 percent aqueous solution of the dye. References to the above reported studies are found in Table III.

The long-term feeding studies on a large group of mice showed no incidence of tumors. A long-term study with 10 rats was also negative for tumors. However, the reports of these studies lack data on histopathological examinations and on chemical and biochemical properties. Consequently, no evaluation was made (333).

The Scientific Committee for Food of the Commission of the European Communities endorsed the decision not to establish an acceptable daily intake for man for this colorant because of the inadequacy of the available data, and it stated that in the committee's opinion this color was not acceptable for use in food (334).

No reviews on the toxicology of this compound but three reviews on its specifications (335,336,337) are available. Analytical aspects are found in reference 338. Some information is also found in reference 339.

FAST YELLOW AB

This monoazo compound has been classified in the category of colorants for which the available toxicological data were inadequate for evaluation and for which virtually no information on long-term toxicity was available (329,340). The toxicological evidence on which this decision was based is partially found in references 341 and 342.

Following oral administration to rats, unchanged dye was found in urine (1 percent of total), and bile (5 percent of total), but none was found in feces. The products of azo-reduction, sulfanilic a id, and p-phenylenediamine sulfonic acid were excreted in urine (57 percent and 6 percent of the total dose, respectively) and in feces, in addition to the acetylated conjugates of these metabolites. Oral administration of these metabolites resulted in 53 percent or 19 percent of the initial dose in the urine. If given intraperitoneally, the dye was excreted in urine. Of an intravenous dose in rats, 2-16 percent was recovered in bile collected over a six-hour period. In rats, after 5mg of dye labeled with ^{14}C in one benzene ring, given by gavage, radioactivity was highest in liver, kidney, muscle, and blood. No radioactivity was detectable in urine after 24 hours.

Azo-reduction of fast yellow AB occurred under anaerobic conditions with the supernatant fraction from sonically disrupted Streptococcus faecalis. Flavoproteins were implicated in the reduction.

At 200-400 mg/liter, pepsin, but not lipase activity was inhibited. At 0.67 µM, the dye decreased the respiration rate of rat liver homogenates. The dye had no sensitization activity in the guinea-pig and the test for Heinz bodies was negative in the cat. At 0.5 g/100 ml, the dye was negative for mutagenicity in E. coli.

Rat intraperitoneal LD_{50} was in the range of 2 g/kg bw; the intravenous in the range of 2.5-5 g/kg bw and the oral in the range of 10 g/kg bw.

A group of 10 rats was fed this dye at a level of 1 percent of the diet for a period of 188 days. Each animal received approximately 1.1 g/kg per day. The animals were kept under observation for 753 days. No tumors were observed.

Eighty-five rats were fed this color at a level of 0.1 percent of the diet for life. Each animal received from 10 to 15 mg per day. No tumors were observed.

Ten rats were fed this dye at a level of 0.2 percent of the diet for a period of 420 days. The animals received 0.1 g/kg per day. They were kept under observations for 791 days. No tumors were observed.

Eleven rats were given subcutaneous injections twice weekly of 0.5 ml of 2 percent solution (1000 mg) for a period of 365 days, at which time 1 g had been administered. The animals were kept under observations for 1,044 days, but no tumors developed. References to these studies are found in Table III.

Limited metabolic data are available on this compound. The long-term rat-feeding study was deficient in detail and did not permit an adequate assessment; thus no evaluation was made (343). Furthermore, no reproduction studies are available.

The Scientific Committee for Food of the Commission of the European Communities endorsed the decision not to establish an acceptable daily intake for man for this colorant because of the inadequacy of the available data and it stated that in the committee's opinion this color was not acceptable for use in food (334).

No reviews on the toxicology of this compound, are available but two reviews on its specifications (344,345) are. Analytical aspects are found in reference 346. Other information is found in reference 347. It was observed that no source of this food color product could be identified (343).

FERROUS GLUCONATE

Ferrous gluconate, as well as ferrous lactate, is a coloring adjunct which gives black color in the presence of tannins. This property and its use justified the inclusion of ferrous gluconate among the food colors (348). When ingested, ferrous gluconate dissociates into ferrous iron (11) and gluconate ion; the biological and toxicological aspects of iron have been considered (349) and those of gluconic acid as well (350,351).

Ferrous gluconate was evaluated not in relation to its use as a nutritional supplement, but rather as a coloring agent (352).

Although there are no specific short-term or long-term studies available on ferrous gluconate, the knowledge of its conversion into ferrous iron and gluconate ion with the observations from the long-standing therapeutic use of ferrous gluconate in man at doses of 1 g or more per day, constitute a basis for evaluation. An ADI not specified* was allocated to this compound, with the reservation that the contribution from ferrous gluconate to the total dietary gluconic acid intake from all sources should be included in the ADI for man of gluconic acid (50 mg/kg bw) (351,353).

One review on this compound (354) and one on its specifications (355) are available. Analytical aspects are found in reference 356.

---

*See footnote on page 26.

FLUORESCEIN

This xanthene compound was classified in the category of colors for which the available data were inadequate for evaluation, but for which the possibility of harmful effects was indicated. (317,357). The toxicological evidence on which this decision was based is partially found in references 358 and 359. Because of its nephotoxic properties and its possible conversion from erythrosine, the chemical specifications of this latter compound were amended to exclude the presence of fluorescein (360) (see also the profile for erythrosine).

Six rats were orally given 500 mg of the color per kg bw and it was found that 91 percent was excreted after eight days. Intravenous application of 3 mg/kg bw showed in six male rats after two hours excretion via the bile approximately 14 percent (9-19 percent) and in the urine approximately 30 percent (20-40 percent). The data show that basic fluorescein structure is stable in all instances. It is possible that glucuronic acid conjugation occurred.

The rat intraperitoneal LD_{50} is in the range of 600 mg/kg bw; the rabbit intravenous LD_{50} is in the range of 300 mg/kg bw.

This color was tested for mutagenic activity with the disc method. The used concentration was 10^{-4} M, stated to be of the same order of magnitude as that used in foodstuff. Studies with streptomycin-dependent E. coli were also carried out. No mutagenic effect was observed in these bacterial tests.

Rats were given a diet containing 0.25, 0.5, 1.0, 2.0, 5.0, and 0 percent of the color for 90 days. Granulation of the kidneys at 1.0, 2.0, and 5.0 percent dosage levels was the most important observation.

Fifteen albino rats were subjected to subcutaneous injections of 1 ml of a 5 percent aqueous solution of the sodium salt of the color once or twice weekly. Several rats died early without showing tumors at the injection site. Of the 8 rats surviving 245 days or more, receiving 57 injections, sarcomas developed in two and two others had small fibromas at the site of injection. One tumor was transplanted up to the fifth generation. No significant change was noted in internal organs at autopsy. Twenty rats were subjected to subcutaneous injections of 1 ml of a 5 percent suspension of the color in olive oil once or twice weekly. Three rats survived 200 days or more. No tumors were observed. References to these studies are found in Table III.

No reviews on the toxicology of this compound or its specifications are available. Some information is found in reference 368. For limit of fluorescein in erythrosine see reference 361.

FOOD GREEN S

This triarylmethane compound was classified in the category of colors for which the available data are inadequate for evaluation, but for which a substantial amount of detailed information is available concerning results of long-term tests (362,363).

In a subsequent evaluation, it has been observed that this color has been studied in adequate long-term feeding studies in rats and also parenterally in mice, but metabolic studies in several animal species, preferably including man, and two-year studies in a non-rodent mammalian species were necessary. At this time, a temporary acceptable daily intake for man of 5mg/kg bw was allocated, based on a demonstrated no-effect level in the rat (1000 mg/kg bw/day) (364,365).

In a further evaluation, it was noted that this color had been studied in adequate long-term tests in rats. However, metabolic information was lacking and the short-term studies were not adequate for evaluation. No adequate reproduction and embryotoxicity, including teratology studies, were available. Indicated areas for further research comprised metabolic studies in several species preferably including man, studies in a second rodent species, and studies in non-rodent species reproduction and embryotoxicity, including teratology studies. Because of the unavailability of additional data requested in the earlier evaluation, the temporary ADI for man was withdrawn (366,367).

The Scientific Committee for Food of the Commission of the European Communities endorsed the temporary ADI previously established, but departed from the latest decision to withdraw the temporary ADI because this was claimed not to be based on new evidence of toxicity. It was considered that it would not create a risk to the health of the consumer if the period of temporary acceptability of this color for use in food was extended. However, the need was emphasized to provide the results of an adequate long-term study in a second species; metabolic studies in several species and, if possible, in man; and studies on reproduction and embryotoxicity, including teratogenicity. This committee has maintained a temporary ADI for man of 5 mg/kg bw for this color (368).

Three reviews on the toxicology of this compound (369); (wool green BS) (370); (wool green BS) (371); (Green S) and four reviews on its specifications (372); (wool green B) (373); (wool green BS) (374); (food green S) (375); (food green S) are available. Analytical aspects are found in references 376 and 377. Other information is is found in reference 378.

GOLD

Gold as a food coloring agent was considered, but no attempt was made a toxicological evaluation (379,380).

Gold salts are used in the treatment of rheumatoid arthritis and have been associated with numerous side effects such as blood dyscrasia, rashes, gastrointestinal disturbances, and nephropathy. The absorption of gold compounds and their distribution in tissues depends on their aqueous solubility and the route of administration. Most gold compounds are poorly absorbed from the gastrointestinal tract. The distribution of gold has been studied in man and animals and it has been found it is bound primarily to plasma proteins. Excretion of gold salts is primarily via the kidney, but some gold finds its way into the feces. The rate of excretion in the urine does not directly reflect the concentration in the plasma, although it diminishes as the concentration in the plasma drops in any individual subject.

It has been shown that the gold concentrates in the kidneys, primarily in the mitochondria of the proximal tubules, and the number of the mitochondria affected are proportional to the dose. The accumulation of gold destroys the mitochondria and they are expelled into the tubular lumen. After withdrawal of the drug, the tubular structure returns to normal. References to these studies are found in Table III.

Intake of gold from food is limited to the use of this color for surface coloring and decoration of food and in special liqueurs. In view of the rare use of gold as a food colorant and the lack of knowledge of the exact nature of the gold used on or in foods, no chemical specifications were prepared. No data were available on the toxicity of elemental gold. In view of the very small amounts likely to be ingested by an individual, it was not considered that the use of gold in food would present a hazard to the health of the consumer (381).

Because of the inadequacy of the available biological information on metallic gold, the Scientific Committee for Food of the Commission of the European Communities concluded that an ADI for man could not be established. However, the use of metallic gold for surface coloring and decoration of food has been accepted without further investigation (382).

No reviews on the toxicology of this substance or on its specifications are available.

GUINEA GREEN B

This triarylmethane compound was classified in the category of colors found to be harmful and which should not be used in food (329, 379). The toxicological evidence on which this decision was based is partially derived from references 383 and 3.

This color is, like other triarylmethane dyes, reported to be excreted largely unchanged in the feces of rats, indicating that it is poorly absorbed in the intestinal tract. A variety of long-term tests in rats and mice has been carried out. In one of these, lymphosarcomata were observed in two out of nine rats fed this color at a level of 4 percent in the diet. In another study, an increased incidence of skin tumors was recorded in rats fed at a level of 3 percent guinea green B. In a third study, nine rats fed at a level of 5 percent had primary hepatic tumors; two of which were malignant. This compared to none in the control group. Evidence of carcinogenic activity is reported in three separate studies. References to these studies are found in Table III.

In a subsequent evaluation of the carcinogenic potential of this compound, it was observed that guinea green B has been tested in mice and rats by oral administration, and in rats by ambient exposure and subcutaneous injection. It was carcinogenic in rats, producing hepatic tumors after its oral administration, local sarcomas after subcutaneous injection, and benign mammary tumors following ambient exposure (384).

One review on the toxicology of this compound (385) and one on its specifications (386) are available. Information is also found in reference 383.

INDANTHRENE BLUE RS

This anthraquinone compound was classified in the category of colors for which the available data were inadequate for evaluation, and for which virtually no information on long-term toxicity was available. Colors for which only long-term studies for tumor formation, unaccompanied by other long-term studies, were considered as falling within this category (379,380).

In a subsequent evaluation, results of long-term studies provided justification for including this color in the category of food colors for which the available data were inadequate for evaluation, but for which a substantial amount of information was available concerning results of long-term tests (387).

In view of these long-term studies, a temporary acceptable daily intake for man (ADI) of 1 mg/kg bw was established, based on a demonstrated no-effect level in the rat (500 mg/kg bw/day) and metabolic studies in several animal species, preferably including man. Two-year studies in a non-rodent mammalian species and long-term studies in the rat of another species were requested (388,389).

In a further evaluation, it was observed that the available long-term study in rats was not adequate, since only some selected parameters had been examined. However, the study provided useful information and did not indicate carcinogenic potential. There was no information on metabolism or on the effects of the color on reproduction, embryotoxicity, and teratogenicity. Because of the unavailability of additional data requested in the earlier evaluation, the temporary ADI for this color was withdrawn (366,390).

The Scientific Committee for Food of the Commission of the European Communities endorsed this decision and it expressed the opinion that this color was not acceptable for use in food (391).

Three reviews on the toxicology of this compound (392,393,394) and two on its specifications (395,396) are available. Analytical aspects are found in reference 397. Other information is found in reference 398.

INDIGOTINE

This indigoid compound had previously been classified in the category of food colors for which the available data were not entirely sufficient to meet the requirements for establishing an acceptable daily intake for man (ADI) (379,380).

In a subsequent evaluation of this color, a temporary ADI for man of 2.5 mg/kg bw was allocated to it, based on a demonstrated no-effect level in the rat (500 mg/kg bw/day) (399,400). At that time, a two-year study in a non-rodent mammalian species was requested (400).

In a further evaluation, an ADI for man of 5 mg/kg bw was allocated to the color based on the no-effect level previously demonstrated in the rat. The toxicological evidence from the newly available information permitted the use of a smaller safety factor (401,402).

The production of a high percentage of local sarcomas at the site of subcutaneous injections in rats, in the past led to considerable discussion and, consequently, to extensive studies on this color and the special conditions of the experiments These studies do not show evidence of carcinogenicity when taken orally. Several species have been investigated in short-term studies; long-term studies in the rat and mouse are available. The metabolic studies on this color are fairly complete and the two long-term studies in the rat do not point to any significant toxic effects. Similarly, a 13-week study on the major metabolite, isatin-5-sulfonic acid, revealed no toxic effects (403).

The Scientific Committee for Food of the Commission of the European Communities endorsed this ADI and it classified this color in the category of food colors for which an ADI could be established and which are, therefore, toxicologically acceptable for use in food within the limits of the ADI (404).

Three reviews on the toxicology of this compound (405,406,407) and three on its specifications (405,408,409) are available. Analytical aspects are found in references 410 and 411. Other information is found in reference 412.

IRON OXIDES (AND HYDRATED IRON OXIDES)

These inorganic compounds are powders also available as mixtures. They occur in various colors, ranging from yellow to orange to black. The principal compounds comprise hydrated iron (III) oxides, iron (III) oxide (iron sesquioxide), iron (II, III) oxide (II, III) oxide (413).

Iron is a vital component of the body. Over 70 percent of the body's iron is normally present as hemoglobin, 3 percent as myoglobin, and 16 percent as transport iron. Iron may be stored in two forms by the organism: as a ferritin (an iron-protein complex) and as hemosiderin. There has been no toxicological investigation of the various iron oxides and hydroxides used as coloring agents in animals or in man by oral administration.

There are, however, many studies on the inhalation, intratracheal, subcutaneous, and intramuscular route, as well as on the muscular route, in relation to the potential carcinogenic effect of iron ore dust and hematite dust. These studies are not pertinent to the evaluation of iron oxides and hydroxide pigments as food colors. Despite the extensive knowledge of the physiological and pharmaceutical effects of other forms of iron, the data cannot be extrapolated specifically to these compounds; each must be evaluated in its own context and consideration given to the problem of haemosiderosis. A temporary ADI not specified* has been allocated to these substances, because of absence of information on physiological absorption and storage of iron, following the use of these pigments as food colorants (414,415).

Indicated areas for required research comprise adequate data on the absorption and storage of iron following use of these pigments (415).

In a subsequent evaluation, the need for human absorption studies was reaffirmed and the previously established ADI was extended (40). Three separate specifications were prepared for the three iron oxides; yellow (hydrated ferric oxide), black (ferrous-ferric oxide), and red (anhydrous ferric oxide). Further information was required for the determination of iron in the case of ferrous-ferric oxide and the water-soluble impurities (40,721).

The Scientific Committee for Food of the Commission of the European Communities classified these colors among the food colors for which an ADI could be established and which were, therefore, toxicologically acceptable for use in food within an ADI with no upper limit specified (416).

Two reviews on the toxicology of these substances (417,418) and three on their specifications (419,420,721) are available. Analytical aspects are found in reference 421.

LIGHT GREEN SF

This triarylmethane compound has been classified in the category of food colors for which the available data were inadequate for evaluation, but indicated the possibility of harmful effects (422,423), producing more than 10-13 percent of local sarcomas at the site of repeated subcutaneous injections (424).

The coloring properties of light green SF were reported in 1879. It is prepared commercially by condensing ethylbenzylaniline with benzaldehyde followed by sulphonation and oxidation, and finally, conversion to the sodium salt. In the past, it was primarily used in food and drugs for coloring products such as gelatin desserts, maraschino cherries, ice creams and sherbets, sweets and confections, bakery products and cereals, and gelatine capsules for pharmaceutical preparations; however, it is no longer believed to be used in these applications. Light green SF is not included in the list of colorants permitted for use in foods in the European Economic Communities; however, it may provisionally be used in cosmetics which come into contact with mucous membranes (425).

This color has been tested in mice and rats by oral administration, and in rats by subcutaneous and intraperitoneal injection. It is carcino-

---

*See note on page 26.

genic in rats after its subcutaneous injection, producing local sarcomas (426).

No acceptable daily intake for man (ADI) has been established for this colorant. References to available toxicological studies are found in Table III.

One review on the toxicology of this compound (427) and two reviews on its specifications (428,429) are available. Analytical aspects are found in reference 397. Other information is found in reference 430.

LITHOL RUBINE BK

This monoazo compound was classified in the category of food colors for which the available data were inadequate for evaluation, and for which virtually no information on long-term toxicity was available. Colorants with long-term studies were considered as falling within this category (380,422).

Data on acute toxicity in the rat and dog are available as well as on dermal toxicity. Groups of five female and five male rats were fed diets containing the color at dosage levels of 0, 0.25, 0.5, 1.0, and 2.0 for 18 weeks. No abnormalities in food intake, body weight, blood counts, organ weights, and histopathology were observed. In long-term studies in the rat, at 2 percent level, slight lower body weight in males was observed. In a study on the dog, 1 percent in the diet caused a change in thryoid weight in males with no associated pathology.

Groups of 10 pregnant rabbits received suspensions of D+C Red No. 7 by stomach tube at doses of 50, 16, and 5 mg/kg/day from day six through day 18 of gestation. On the basis of number of viable and dead fetuses; resorption sites; mean fetal weight; distribution by sex, mean litter size; frequency of skeletal, visceral or structural anomalies; weight gain of pregnant females; D+C Red No. 7 evidenced no effect on reproductive performance, maternal weight gain, and fetal development.

Groups of 20 pregnant rats received suspensions of D+C Red No. 7 by stomach tube at doses of 50, 16, and 5 mg/kg/day from day six through day 15 of gestation. On the basis of a number of viable and dead fetuses; resorption sites; mean fetal weight distribution by sex; mean litter size; frequency of skeletal visceral or structural anomalies, weight gain of pregnant females; D+C Red No. 7 was without effect on reproductive performance, maternal weight gain, and fetal development. However, mink fed cheese rind containing lithol rubin had reduced litter number.

Groups of rats (10 male and 20 female per group) were given lithol rubin BCA mixed in their diet to provide daily doses of 50.0, 15.0, 5, or 0.5 mg/kg bw/day. The parent generation rats were bred twice; the Flb were bred three times and the F2b were bred once. The criteria of effect measured included fertility; gestation; gestation survival; four-day, 14-day, and 21-day survivals; diet consumption and body weights of the parent rats and their progeny; number of resorption sites; and corpore lutea at the 19-day kill of the 3rd mating of the Flb parents. The 50.0 mg/kg rats in the second generation had lower fertility indexes than did their controls. This condition was neither present at 50.0 mg/kg in the third generation nor at 15.0 mg/kg in any generation. In the order criteria, the differences in the three generations of reproduction of rats between dosed and control groups were either not dosage-related, not progressive, or were indicative of mean or median values exceeding those of the controls. References to these studies are found in Table III. No acceptable daily intake for man to this colorant was allocated (431).

The Scientific Committee for Food of the Commission of the European Communities classified this color among these for which an ADI could not

be established, but which are nevertheless acceptable for external coloring of cheese rind only. It requested results of migration studies; metabolic studies in animals and, if possible, in man; and long-term
studies in two animal species, because it had been informed that deli-
berate ingestion of cheese rind containing this coloring matter had become a practice (432).

No review on the toxicology and only one review on its specifications (433) is available. Analytical aspects are found in reference 434.

LYCOPENE

This natural carotenoid contained in tomato extracts underwent
trials as red food coloring to replace, to an increasing extent, red
azo dyes. However, lack of information on this carotenoid derived both
from natural and synthetic sources prevented a toxicological assessment
(435).

In a subsequent examination, it was observed that no manufacturer
of lycopene as a food color was known. Data were available on an un-
specified material consisting of a single-generation reproduction study
and a short-term study in the rat. These studies were considered to be
inadequate from the point of view of the number of animals and the factors examined; thus no evaluation could be made (436). Reference to the
above mentioned studies is found in Table III.

Without further investigations, the Scientific Committee for Food
of the Commission of the European Communities classified lycopene, prepared from natural foods by physical processes, among colors for which
an ADI could not be established, but which are nevertheless acceptable
for use in food generally (437).

No review on the toxicology of this substance and no review on its
specifications are available.

MAGENTA

This triarylmethane compound has been classified in the category of
food colors found to be harmful and which should not be used in food
(438,439). The toxicological evidence on which this decision has been
based is derived from reference 3. References to the studies contained
in this document are found in Table III.

Although the quantity consumed is probably quite small, magenta is
widely used in medicine as a microbiological stain. One source has described the basic fuchsines (magenta and related dyes) as among the most
powerful nuclear dyes and has listed 26 biological stains in which they
are used. Magenta has been reported to be used for meat-marking colors
in New Zealand.

The grade of magenta used in medicine, basic fuchsin NF, is approved
for use in carbol-fuchsin solution NF, an antifungal agent containing
phenol and resorcinol. No evidence is available to indicate that this
solution is presently being used in the U.S., but it is probably used
elsewhere (440).

In a recent evaluation of the potential for carcinogenicity of this
compound, it was observed that the only evidence for the carcinogenicity
of magenta is the induction of local sarcomas in rats following subcutaneous administration of para-magenta, one of the components of commercial magenta. This positive result has been due to the physical, rather
than to the chemical properties of this substance. Oral administration
of the commercial product to mice produced negative effects in a single
study, but the finding was based upon an insufficient number of surviv-

ing animals. One epidemiological study appears to establish the carcinogenic risk to workers involved in the manufacture of this substance. On
present evidence, it is not possible to indicate whether the industrial
bladder cancer found in workers is attributable to the exposure to magenta itself, or to one or more of its associated intermediates and impurities (441).

One review on the toxicology of this compound (442) and none on its
specifications is available. Some information is also found in reference
443.

MALACHITE GREEN

This triarylmethane compound has been classified in the category
of food colors for which the available data were inadequate for evaluation, but which indicate the possibility of harmful effects (438,439).
The toxicological evidence on which this decision has been based is derived from reference 444.

The oral LD_{50} in the mouse is in the range of 20 to 750 mg/kg bw;
the intravenous, in the range of 100 mg; the intraperitoneal, in the
range of 4.2 mg; and the intravenous in the rat in the range of 30-35
mg/kg bw. In the rat, this color gives a clear change of the electro-
cardiogram.

Groups of 10 males and 10 females were fed diets containing 0, 0.03,
0.3, and 3.0 percent of the color for 64 weeks. The rats fed 0.3 and
3.0 percent died all within one week. At the end of the experiment, there
was no significant difference in mortality in the group of 0.03 percent
and the control group. The female rats fed the color showed a significant decrease in food intake and in growth rate throughout the experiment. There was a significant increase in the relative liver weight of
these animals compared to the controls. No histopathological abnormalities were found.

A group of rats, five males and five females, was given the color
in their drinking water for about six months and, after this period,
the color was given intermittently by stomach tube. The offspring of
these animals, which were not treated with the color, showed various
disturbances up to the 12th untreated generation. The following effects
were observed: (1) disturbances indicating changes in the hereditary
pattern (abnormalities in the bones, eyes, skin, lungs, and teratogenic
effects. Also, sterility was found). (2) marked frequency of various
tumors in different organs (lung, mammary, and ovary).

A group of animals treated in the same way, but also given cyto-
chrome C simultaneously with the color, did not show these abnormalities.
The control group, three males and three females, did not show any pathological symptoms.

Another experiment was carried out in the same way described above,
with the only change being that only two to three generations were bred.
The same abnormalities were found.

From transplantation studies, it was found that the mammary tumors
were malignant. The transplantation succeeds more easily on the offspring
of rats originally injured with the color than on control animals. References to these studies are found in Table III.

These studies are difficult to evaluate because they were performed
on animals each treated individually, and the quantities of color and
duration of treatment are not stated.

No review on the toxicology of this compound or on its specifications
is available. Some information is found in reference 445.

METHANIL YELLOW

This monoazo compound has been classified in the category of food colors for which the available data were inadequate for evaluation, and for which virtually no information on long-term toxicity was available. Colors with long-term tests for tumor formation, unaccompanied by other long-term studies, were considered as falling within this category (438, 439).

The toxicological evidence on which this decision was based is derived from reference 446.

The oral LD_{50} in the mouse was estimated at 5 g/kg bw; the intravenous, 0.2 g/kg bw. Thirty mice were fed 15-20 mg per week of metanil yellow for periods up to 835 days. No tumors or liver lesions were observed. References to these studies are found in Table III.

No review of the toxicology of this compound or on its specifications is available. Some information is found in reference 447.

METHYL VIOLET

This triarylmethane compound has been classified in the category of food colors for which the available data were inadequate for evaluation, and for which virtually no information on long-term toxicity was available. Colors with long-term tests for tumor formation, unaccompanied by other long-term studies, were considered as falling within this category (438,448).

The Scientific Committee for Food of the Commission of the European Communities considered methyl violet as a mixture of the hydrochlorides of the more highly methylated pararosaniline containing principally tetramethyl, pentamethyl and hexamethyl derivatives. On the bas s of the very scanty acute toxicity data available, which did not include any result of tests by the oral route, it was not possible to arrive at an evaluation of this color. Data were available indicating that the only current use of methyl violet is as a marker (e.g. for meat, citrus fruit). It was recommended that this substance should not be used to color food and that its use as a marker should be reconsidered (723).

No review on the toxicology of this compound, but one review on its specifications is available (449). Some information is found in reference 450.

NAPHTHOL BLUE BLACK

This disazo compound has been classified in the category of food colors for which the available data were inadequate for evaluation, and for which virtually no information on long-term toxicity was available. Colors with long-term tests for tumor formation, unaccompanied by other long-term studies, were considered as falling within this category (438, 439). The toxicological evidence on which this decision was based is partially derived from reference 451.

No data are available on biochemical aspects or acute toxicity. Only a short-term study in the rat has been carried out.

Five groups of 20 rats each were fed the color for 90 days at dosage levels of 0.25, 0.5, 1.0, and 2.0 percent. In both sexes and at all dosage levels, the mean weight gain was less than the controls, and the mean weights of the spleens were larger than the controls at all levels, but not statistically significant. Only two animals on the 2.0 percent level survived 90 days. Reference to this study is found in Table III.

No review on the toxicology of this compound or on its specifications is available. Some information is found in reference 452.

NAPHTHOL YELLOWS

This nitro compound was classified in the category of food colors for which the available data were inadequate for evaluation, but which indicated the possibility of harmful effects (438,439). The toxicological evidence on which this decision was based has not been published in the form of a monograph, but can partially be derived from reference 453.

A total of 96 male and female mice, produced by mixed breeding from five different strains, were given a diet containing 1 mg per animal per day of the food color. Mice at the age of 50-100 days were used. A number of the animals were sacrificed after an observation period of 500 days and the rest of the survivors after 700 days. A total of 168 mice were used as negative controls. Positive control groups which were given o-aminoazo-toluene and dimethylaminoazobenzene, were also included. In these groups, the formation of liver tumors was noted after approximately 200 days. The incidence of tumors in mice receiving the dye was not significantly greater than in the negative controls. It was concluded that this color had no carcinogenic action.

This color in a concentration of 60 mg/liter inhibited the action of pepsin, but lipase action was not affected. The dye was fed at a level of 0.1 percent of the diet to 85 rats for 200 days. Each animal ingested 10 to 15 mg per day. No tumors were observed.

Intraperitoneal LD_{50} in mice was found to be in the order of 150 mg/kg bw. An oral dose of 1 g/kg bw produced no effect in five mice. In a 20-week feeding experiment, all five rats died at a dosage level of 1 percent.

Dosage levels of 100 and 1000 ppm produced no effect in rats in two-year experiments. In a five-year experiment, 100 mg/kg/day produced no effect in two dogs and 5 mg/kg/day produced no effects in three dogs.

Chronic feeding studies have been recently completed with rats; however, histopathological examination of the tissues of these animals is just beginning. In a two-year feeding experiment, this dye was fed at dosage levels of 2, 1, 0.5, 0.25, and 0.1 percent. All animals in the two highest levels died within a year. The outstanding gross effect was extensive ulceration in the cecum and terminal colon at the three highest levels (2,1, and 0.5 percent), with a trace of the effect at 0.25 percent. Slight or moderate splenic enlargement frequently accompanied the more pronounced degrees of gut ulceration. References to these studies are found in Table III.

No review on the toxicology of this compound but one review on its specifications in available (454. Some information is also found in reference 453.

NIGROSINE

This hydroxyketone compound was classified in the category of food colors for which the available information was not adequate for evaluation, but indicated the possibility of harmful effects (438,439). The evidence for this decision is partially found in an unpublished document (455) and in reference 456.

The intravenous LD_{50} in the rat was found to be in the range of 200 mg/kg bw. Two groups of 10 rats were given 0.5 percent of the color in drinking water for 402 and 465 days, respectively. The total intake of the color was about 50 g per animal in both groups. The observation period was 545 days. One animal died within this time. No tumors were found.

Four groups of 20 rats (10 female and 1ᵥ male) were given diets containing 0.0, 0.03, 0.3, and 3.0 percent of the color for 64 weeks. The female rats with a 3.0 percent diet showed a significant decrease in growth rate. In both male and female rats receiving the diet with 3 percent, an increase in the organ body weight ratio for liver and kidneys was observed. In the kidney and testis, histopathological lesions were found; but not in the liver.

One rat was given twice weekly subcutaneous injections of 0.5 ml of a 1 percent solution of the color for 42 days. The total dose injected was 60 mg. The observation period was 522 days. This animal showed a sarcoma at the site of injection.

One cat was given 0.1 g of the color per kg body weight orally for seven days. No Heinz bodies were found.

A total of 117 mice, 70 male and 47 female, produced by mixed breeding from five different strains, were given a diet containing 1 mg per animal per day of the color. Mice between the ages of 50 to 100 days were used. A number of the animals were sacrificed after an observation period of 500 days, and the rest of the survivors after 700 days. A total of 168 mice were used as a negative control. Positive control groups, which were given o-aminoazo-toluene and dimethylaminoazobenzene, were also included. In these groups, the formation of liver tumors was noted after approximately 200 days. The incidence of tumors in mice receiving the color to be tested was not significantly greater than in the controls.

Twenty rats were given twice weekly subcutaneous injections of 0.5 ml of a 0.25 percent solution of the color for 16 weeks. The total dose injected was 40 mg per animal. The observation period was 577 days. Sarcomas were found in five animals at the site of injection.

Ten rats were given twice weekly subcutaneous injections of 0.5 ml of a 1 percent solution of the color for 25 days. The total dose injected was 20 mg per animal. The observation period was 808 days. No tumors were found.

Two rats were given subcutaneous injections of 0.5 ml of a 1 percent solution of the color twice weekly for 25 days. The total dose injected was 40 mg. The observation period was 768 days. In the two animals, no tumors were found at the site of injection. This color contains a variety of amines and nitroso compounds. Sarcomas have been produced as a result of subcutaneous injections.

References to these studies are found in Table III.

No review on the toxicology of this compound or on its specifications is available. Information can be found in reference 456.

OIL ORANGE SS

This monoazo color was first synthesized in 1878. In 1972, only one U.S. manufacturer reported production of it. There may be as many as five producers of oil orange SS in Western Europe, but current production is believed to be small. In 1972, there were believed to be four Japanese producers, who manufactured 4,100 kg of this color.

This substance has been approved for use as a general food coloring in Canada, Greece, Japan, Mexico, New Zealand, Norway, Peru, and South Africa, Subsequent reports indicate that it has been approved also in Cuba, the Dominican Republic, Guatemala, and Venezuela. Approval had been withdrawn in Canada, New Zealand, and Norway. Approval for its use in food was withdrawn in Japan prior to 1966; however, it is permitted for certain non-food uses.

Oil orange SS was added to the U.S. approved list of food, drug, and cosmetic colors, however, on the basis of toxicological data, it was removed from the list for use in food, but was permitted in externally applied drugs and cosmetics. It was later removed for even these uses (457).

This substance has been classified as a color found to be harmful and which should not be used in food (438,439). The toxicological evidence on which this decision was based is derived from references 3 and 458. References to these studies are found in Table III.

The carcinogenic potential of this substance has been more recently examined when it was observed that oil orange SS is carcinogenic in mice following its oral and subcutaneous administration, producing intestinal and local tumors; it also produced carcinomas of the bladder in mice following its administration by bladder implantation. Tests by the oral and subcutaneous routes in rats were either inadequately reported or of too short duration to be evaluated (459).

One review on the toxicology of this compound (460) and no review on its specifications is available. Information is also found in reference 458.

OIL ORANGE XO

In 1972, three U.S. manufacturers reported production of this monoazo color. In Western Europe, there may be as many as eight producers; one producer in the United Kingdom manufactures some several thousand kg per year. In Japan, three producers manufactured 3,300 kg of this color in 1972 (461).

This substance has been approved for use as a general food coloring in Canada, Greece, Japan, Mexico, Norway, and Peru. Subsequent reports indicated that it has also been approved in Cuba, the Dominican Republic, and Guatemala and that its approval for use in food has been withdrawn in Canada and Norway. Approval for its use in food in Japan was subsequently withdrawn, although it was retained for certain nonfood uses.

The color was added to the U.S. approved list of food, drug, and cosmetic colors, but subsequently, on the basis of toxicological findings, was removed from this list for use in food, but permitted in externally applied drugs and cosmetics. It was later removed even for these uses (462).

This compound has been classified as a color found to be harmful, and which should not be used in food (438,463). The toxicological evidence on which this decision was based is derived from references 3 and 464. Reference to the studies reported in these documents is found in Table III.

The carcinogenic potential of this color has been more recently examined when it was observed that oil orange XO was tested in mice and rats by the oral and subcutaneous routes, and that the results of these studies could not be evaluated because of the inadequacy of the number of animals used, the duration of the experiment, or the degree of reporting. This color was also tested in mice by bladder implantation, resulting in a high incidence of bladder carcinomas (465). One review on the toxicology of this compound (466)* and no review on its specifications are available. Information can also be found in reference 467.

_____

*This reference erroneously reports this compound as Sudan II; alternative name is Sudan Red II.

OIL YELLOW AB

This monoazo color was first prepared in 1885. No commercial production in the U.S. has been reported since 1960. In Western Europe, there may be as many as four producers, but production is believed to be small. Several companies in Japan probably manufactured it prior to 1967, when production was believed to have been stopped.

Yellow AB was approved for food use in the U.S., and was subsequently used to color margarine, both in the U.S. and Japan. It has also been reportedly approved for use as a general food coloring in Australia, Canada, Greece, Japan, Mexico, New Zealand, Norway, Peru, South Africa, and the U.S. Additional approvals were reported by Costa Rica, Cuba, Guatemala, and the Philippines, but indications were that approval had been withdrawn in New Zealand and Norway. It was used in France to color margine. In 1959, yellow AB was removed from the U.S. approved list for use in foods, but was permitted in externally applied drugs and cosmetics; in 1960 it was removed completely from the approved list. Approval for its use in food in Japan was withdrawn in 1966, although approval was retained for certain non-food uses (468).

This compound has been classified as a color found to be harmful, and which should not be used in food (438,463). The toxicological evidence on which this decision was based is derived from reference 3 and 469. References to the studies reported in these documents are found in Table III.

Although extensive toxicological studies on oil yellow AB have been carried out, data on the metabolic rate of the color in animals and man are lacking. In various short-term studies, the feeding of from 10 mg/week up to 4 percent of the diet to rats resulted in severe toxic symptoms and deaths in a period of about two months. Toxicity was manifested as stunted growth; marked blood changes; changes in testes, spleen, kidney, and liver; as well as marked increase in mortality. There was no tumor production in mice by skin painting of 0.3 percent dye in benzene for 464 days or by intubation of 1 mg in 0.25 ml of butter or margarine for 403 days. Although quite toxic, the substance was not found to be carcinogenic in this study. It was toxic to dogs above a dietary level of 0.05 percent (500 ppm). One death, and toxic symptoms occurred at a dietary level of 1,000 ppm (0.1 percent).

Long-term studies in rats by several investigators indicate considerable toxicity and increased mortality rate by feeding at various dietary levels. Levels of 0.03 percent (300 ppm) caused slight changes in kidney and liver weight; 8-12 mg/day (equivalent to 400 to 600 ppm in the diet) in a rice diet caused weight losses and increased mortality. Higher levels resulted in severe toxicity to the blood and many of the major organs plus a marked increase in mortality. In spite of the toxicity of oil yellow AB, the dye has not been considered tumorigenic by the oral route and questionable by the subcutaneous route. The only human studies performed were sensitization patch tests which were demonstrated to be positive.

In long-term studies, a non-effect level had not been established. Furthermore, this color displays a variety of toxic effects even at low dietary levels and in practice; it has been found difficult to manufacture a form free of β-naphthylamine, a known carcinogen in man (3, 469).

The carcinogenic potential of this color has been more recently examined when it was observed that oil yellow AB was tested by the oral route in rats and by subcutaneous injections in mice and rats, and the substance was not found to be carcinogenic in these studies (468).

One review on the toxicology of this compound (470)* and no review on its specifications are available. Information is also found in reference 469.

OIL YELLOW OB

This lipid-soluble monoazo color was first prepared in 1905. No production has been reported from the U.S. since 1960. In Western Europe, there may be one producer, but production is believed to be small. Several companies in Japan probably manufactured this color prior to 1967, when its production is believed to have been stopped. It was approved for food use in the U.S. in 1918 and it was subsequently used to color margarine. Approved use for food in general is reported in countries including Australia, Canada, Greece, Japan, Mexico, New Zealand, Norway, Peru, South Africa, and the U.S. Additional approvals were subsequently reported in Costa Rica, Cuba, Guatemala, and the Philippines. Approvals were withdrawn in New Zealand and Norway. It is believed that the color was also used in foodstuffs in Denmark, Finland, and the United Kingdom prior to 1960. It was used in France between April 1947 and October 1958 to color margarine. In 1959, it was removed from the U.S. approved list for use in foods, but was permitted in externally applied drugs and cosmetics; and in 1960 it was removed entirely from the list. Approval for its use in food in Japan was withdrawn in 1966, although approval was retained for certain non-food uses; prior to that time, it had been used to color margarine, oil products, and spirits (471).

This compound has been classified as a color found to be harmful, and which should not be used in food (438,463). The toxicological evidence on which this decision was based is derived from references 3 and 472. References to the studies reported in these documents are found in Table III.

In a long-term study in rats and a short-term study in dogs, a no-effect level was indicated at 500 ppm, but pathological changes including cardiac hypertrophy were noted at levels of 1,000 ppm and above. In a 65-week test on rats, diets containing 300 ppm resulted in increased liver and kidney weight and a decrease in the weight of testes. Tumor incidence after oral dosage was not demonstrated, but the compound was mildly carcinogenic when injected subcutaneously. The compound undergoes metabolism in the stomach of the rabbit. In practice, it has been found difficult to produce this color in a form free from B-naphthylamine (3,472).

The carcinogenic potential of this color has been more recently examined when it was observed that oil yellow OB had been tested in mice by subcutaneous injection and in rats by oral and subcutaneous administration. Although the feeding experiments in rats and the subcutaneous injection studies in mice were negative, the color produced local tumors in rats, following its subcutaneous administration (473).

One review on the toxicology of this compound (474)** and no review on its specifications are available. Some information is also found in reference 472.

---

*This reference reports this compound as yellow AB.
**This reference reports this compound as yellow OB.

OLEORESIN OF PAPRIKA

This natural coloring and flavoring agent is the product obtained by solvent extraction of the pods of <u>Capsicum annum L.</u>, with the subsequent removal of the solvent. It contains capsaicin ($C_{18}H_{27}NO_3$), a carotenoic pigment. It appears as a deep red somewhat viscid liquid with characteristic odor and peppery (hot) taste. Article of commerce may also be specified for its color value. The color imparted to a food product can range from a deep crimson red to a pale pinkish-yellow, depending on the concentrations used. It is also used in combination with annatto to color processed cheese. This oleoresin consists of about 37 to 54 pigments, depending on the mode of preparation (extract of unbleached or bleached paprika), of which only 21 and 33 respectively could be completely or even tentatively identified. The main pigments are in general esters of capsanthin and capsorubin. Most assay methods, therefore, are based on the determination of these two carotenoids (475).

The active principal capsaicin has systemic and local irritant action. The effect observed in a short-term study in rats on a grossly sub-normal diet is not relevant to an evaluation for human use (476).

The use of the oleoresin as a spice is self-limiting and obviates the need for an acceptable daily intake figure (476,477). It may consequently be inferred that the substance has an acceptable daily intake "not specified"*(478).

One review on the toxicology of this substance (476) and one review on its specifications (475) are available.

ORANGE I

This monoazo color was first synthesized in 1876. U.S. production was last reported in 1961, when this color was manufactured by one company. In Western Europe, there may have been as many as 11 producers of Orange I in the past, but it is believed that present production is small. The production of this color in Japan was stopped in 1966.

This color was one of the seven original colors permitted under the U.S. Pure Food and Drugs Act of 1906, and it was reported early as approved for use as a general food coloring in many countries throughout the world; known exceptions at that time were the Federal Republic of Germany, Finland, Spain, Turkey, The United Kingdom, the USSR, and Yugoslavia. Latter reports indicate that it was not permitted in Bulgaria, Canada, Denmark, India, the Netherlands, New Zealand, Norway, Portugal, South Africa, Sweden, or the U.S. In Japan, approval for its use in food was withdrawn prior to 1966, although it was retained for certain non-food uses. It was removed from the approved list for food use in the U.S. in 1956, but was permitted in externally applied drugs and cosmetics; however, in 1968, approval for these latter uses was also discontinued, on the basis of toxicological evidence (479).

Toxicological experiments have been carried out in three animal species; however, no satisfactory no-effect levels have been demonstrated. Since data were insufficient to permit a toxicological assessment of this compound, no ADI for man has been allocated to it (480,481, 482,483).

It appears that no manufacturer produces this color for food use any longer. Summaries of short-term studies on this compound in several animal species were reviewed. These studies were carried out at dose

---

*See footnote on page 26.

levels that produced toxic effects. Summaries of long-term studies in rats and mice, and short-term studies in dogs were available. However, it was not possible to demonstrate a no-effect level in any of these studies. Thus, it was not possible to establish an acceptable daily intake for man (483).

In an evaluation of the carcinogenic potential of this compound, it was observed that this color has been tested by the oral route in mice, rats, and dogs, but the studies could not be evaluated due to inadequate reporting. It was also tested by the subcutaneous route in rats, producing injection site tumors (484).

Four reviews on the toxicology of this compound (23,485,486,487) and one review on its specifications (488) are available. Some information is also found in reference 489.

ORANGE II

This monoazo compound has been classified in the category of food colors for which the available data were inadequate for evaluation and for which no information on long-term toxicity was available. Colors with long-term tests for tumor formation, unaccompanied by other long-term studies, were considered as falling within this category (438, 439). References to some studies are found in Table III.

No review on the toxicology of this compound and no review on its specifications are available. Some information is found in reference 490.

ORANGE G

This monoazo color was first synthesized in 1878. In 1972, eight manufacturers reported production of 131,000 kg in the U.S. In Western Europe, there may be as many as 19 producers of orange G, and it is believed that current annual production is in the order of several hundred thousand kg. In Japan, in 1973, two manufacturers produced approximately 19,000 kg of the color.

In the U.S. this color was used as a drug and cosmetic colorant until October 1966, when its use for these applications was cancelled. Its use in cosmetics was reported to be permitted in the Federal Republic of Germany. It has been reported that it was approved for use in food coloring in Belgium, the German Democratic Republic, Norway, South Africa, Sweden, and the United Kingdom. A later report indicates additional approvals in Australia, Bulgaria, Denmark, and Uruguay; and more recently it has been reported that Denmark, South Africa, and the United Kingdom still use it as a general purpose food color (491).

This color was classified in the category of food colors for which the available data were inadequate, or for which virtually no information on long-term toxicity was available; consequently, no ADI for man could be allocated (438,492).

More recently, the carcinogenic potential of this color has been evaluated and it was observed that orange G was tested only in mice and rats by the oral route. The available studies in mice did not allow an evaluation of the carcinogenic potential of this compound, since in one study the adequacy of the dose could not be assessed, and in the other, information on pathology and survival rates was insufficient. The study in rats could not be evaluated due to limited reporting (493).

The Scientific Committee on Food of the Commission of the European Communities endorsed the decision of not establishing an acceptable daily intake for man because of the inadequacy of the available data, and it classified this color among those food colors for which an ADI could not be established, and which are not toxicologically acceptable for use in food (494).

One review on the toxicology of this compound (495) and one on its specifications (496) are available. Some information is also found in reference 497. Analytical aspects can be found in reference 397.

ORANGE GGN

This monoazo compound was classified in the category of food colors for which the available data were inadequate for evaluation, and for which virtually no information on long-term toxicity was available. Colors with long-term tests for tumor formation unaccompanied by other long-term studies were considered as falling within this category (438, 498). The evidence on which this decision was based can be derived from an unpublished document (3) and reference 499.

In subsequent evaluations, it was not possible to establish an acceptable daily intake for man (ADI) because of the incomplete nature of data available. Long-term studies in the rat have been carried out with this substance, but the published data were lacking in detail and, consequently, were found to be inadequate for toxicological evaluation. Furthermore, no current food additive use was known. The metabolic data on this compound are not adequate and the long-term studies are only concerned with mortality and tumor incidence. No histopathological, biochemical, or hematological information was collected, nor were organ weights examined. The reproduction studies in the rat do not point out any observable effect, however they are lacking detailed observations (00,501).

The Scientific Committee for Food of the Commission of the European Communities endorsed the decision not to establish an acceptable daily intake for man (ADI) because of the inadequacy of toxicological data, and it classified this color among the food colors for which an ADI for man could not be established, and which are not toxicologically acceptable for use in food (494).

One review on the toxicology of this compound (23), and two reviews on its specifications (502,503) are available. Some information is also found in reference 499. Analytical aspects can be found in reference 397.

ORANGE RN

This monoazo compound was classified in the category of food colors for which toxicological data were virtually non-existent (438,439).

In subsequent evaluations, it was observed that in the available short- and long-term studies in mice, rats, and pigs, adverse effects in the hemotopoietic system (Heinz bodies formation) and the liver were found. Metabolites of this color include aminophenols and aniline. Evidence of hemolytic anemia in rats and pigs reinforces the significance of the observations of splenomegaly reported in the available long-term studies in the rat and mouse. In addition, bile duct proliferation has been recorded, which was present in a dose-related manner. It was observed that a no-effect level could not be established in the most sensitive species tested and that an adequate multigeneration study ha not been made. Consequently, no ADI for man has been allocated (504,505,506).

Indicated areas for further research comprise metabolic studies, reproduction, and possibly embryotoxicity and teratological studies (504).

The Scientific Committee for Food of the Commission of the European Communities observed that two commercial products appear to exist for this compound, one containing only orange RN, the other containing 85 percent orange RN and 15 percent subsidiary dye. Some of the biological data referred to one product, and some to the other. Therefore, the decision of not establishing an ADI for man was endorsed because of the inadequacy of the available data. This color was classified in the category of food colors for which an ADI could not be established and which are not toxicologically acceptable for use in food (494).

Two reviews on the toxicology of this compound (23,507) and no review on its specifications are available. Some information is also found in reference 508.

ORCHIL/ORCEIN

Orcein is a mixture of red orcein ($C_{28}H_{24}O_7N_2$) a yellow compound ($C_{21}H_{29}NO_5$) and an amorphous product similar to litmus. Orchil is extracted from Orchella seed (various species of Roccella lichens), or from Orchella moss by treatment with ammonia and exposure to air. It contains orcein, orcin, and litmus. Orchil is a thick reddish-purple liquid with a slight ammoniacal odor; orcein is insoluble in water and soluble in ethanol, acetone, acetic acid, and in alkalies (509).

The reports that there was no substantial use of this material as a food additive and the complete lack of information prevented its toxicological assessment (510).

The Scientific Committee for Food of the Commission of the European Communities endorsed the opinion not to establish an ADI for man because of the inadequacy of data, and it classified this color among the food colors for which an ADI for man could not be established and which are not toxicologically acceptable to use in food (494).

No review on the toxicology of this material and one review on its chemical specifications (509) are available; however these specifications are no longer acceptable (510). Some information is also found in reference 511.

PATENT BLUE V

This triarylmethane compound was classified in the category of food colors for which the available data are inadequate for evaluation, but for which a substantial amount of detailed information is available concerning results of long-term tests (438,512).

In a subsequent evaluation, it was observed that metabolic information on this compound was lacking and long-term reproduction studies in the rat did not reveal any significant toxicological effects. However, the corresponding sodium salt, which is not used as food color, showed evidence of considerable surface activity on subcutaneous injection. For this reason, a long-term study in a second animal species was required. A temporary acceptable daily intake for man of 1 mg/kg bw was established based on a demonstrated no-effect level in rat studies (500 mg/kg bw/day (513,514). Further metabolism studies in several species eferably including man; two year studies in a non-rodent mammalian species; and a long-term study in a second species were requested.

In a further evaluation, the temporary ADI for man previously allocated was withdrawn because of the unavailability of additional data requested in the earlier evaluation (515,516).

The Scientific Committee for Food of the Commission of the European Communities departed from the decision of withdrawing the temporary ADI for man and established a temporary ADI for man of 2.5 mg/kg bw, because it was not considered to create a risk to the health of the consumer if the period of temporary acceptability of this color for use in food were extended. However, the need was emphasized to provide the results of an adequate long-term study in a second animal species, and of a short-term study in a non-rodent species, as well as metabolic studies in several species, if possible also in man, and teratogenicity studies (517).

Three reviews on the toxicology of this compound (518,519,520) and four reviews on its specifications (521,522,523,524) are available. Analytical aspects are found in references 525 and 526. Some information is also found in reference 527.

PERSIAN BERRIES

Persian Berries are the seed-bearing fruit of <u>Rhamnus amygdalinus</u>. They contain the glucosides of the coloring matter, rhamnetin ($C_{16}H_{12}O_7$) and a small proportion of rhamnazin ($C_{17}H_{14}O_7$). Rhamnetin is insoluble in water and only sparingly soluble in alcohol; it decomposes above 300°C. Rhamnazin is very sparingly soluble in alcohol; it dissolves in alkaline liquids to form orange-yellow solutions (528).

The complete lack of information prevented the toxicological assessment of this material (438,516) and no evidence was found of any food use of this color (529).

No review on the toxicology of this substance and no review on its specifications is available. Some information is found in reference 528.

PONCEAU 2R (MX)

This monoazo color was first synthesized in 1878. In 1972, three U.S. producers manufactured 17,000 kg of this color.

In Western Europe, there may be as many as 15 producers of ponceau 2R. Total production data are not available, but it is believed that at least several thousand kg per year are manufactured in the United Kingdom. One Japanese manufacturer reported the production of 3,000 kg of this color in 1972 and 4,000 kg in 1973.

Approval for its use in drugs and cosmetics in the U.S. was cancelled in October 1966. In Japan, it is believed to be used in soaps and face lotions, but its use in pills, capsules, and dental creams is prohibited.

It has been reported that ponceau 2R was approved for food use in the following countries: Argentina, Australia, Belgium, Brazil, Chile, Colombia, Denmark, Egypt, France, Italy, Japan, Mexico, New Zealand, Norway, Poland, South Africa, Sweden, Switzerland, and Uruguay, and for limited use in the United Kingdom. A later report indicates additional approvals in Bolivia, Cambodia, Colombia, Lebanon, Morocco, Tunisia, Turkey, the United Kingdom, and Vietnam; but indicates that approval had been withdrawn in New Zealand, Norway, and Sweden. Although the EEC does not recommend the use of ponceau 2R in foodstuffs, it has recently been reported that it is so used, at least in Denmark. Approval for its use in food was withdrawn in Japan prior to 1966, although it was retained for certain non-food uses (530).

This color was classified in the category of food colors for which the available information is inadequate for evaluation, but indicate the possibility of harmful effects; consequently no ADI for man could be allocated (438,531). The evidence on which this decision was based can be partially derived from reference 532.

More recently, the carcinogenic potential of this color was examined and it was observed that ponceau 2R is carcinogenic, producing liver-cell tumors in mice and rats, and possibly intestinal tumors in mice, following its administration by the oral route. A dose-response effect was noted in the mouse and rat studies (533).

One review on the toxicology of this compound (534)* and one review on its specifications (535) are available. Analytical aspects are found in reference 397. Some information is also found in reference 532.

PONCEAU 3R

This monoazo color was first prepared in 1878. The last report of U.S. commercial production was in 1960, when it was produced by four manufacturers. It is not believed to be produced commercially in either Western Europe or Japan at the present time. Ponceau 3R was one of the seven original food colors permitted under the US Food and Drug Act of 1906; however, on the basis of animal toxicity studies, it was removed from the list of approved substances for use in foodstuffs in November 1960, although it was permitted in externally applied drugs and cosmetics. In 1966, it was removed from the list of approved substances altogether.

It has been reported that this material was approved for use as a general food coloring in Australia, Canada, Denmark, France, Greece, Italy, Japan, Mexico, New Zealand, Norway, Peru, Poland, Portugal, Rumania, South Africa, Sweden, Switzerland, Turkey, Venezuela, and Yugoslavia; and for limited use in the United Kingdom. A more recent report indicated additional approvals in Brazil, Costa Rica, Cuba, the Dominican Republic, Guatemala, Israel, Lebanon, Morocco, the Philippines, Tunisia, the United Kingdom, Uruguay, and Vietnam; but it has been indicated that approval had been withdrawn in France, New Zealand, Norway, Sweden, Switzerland, and Yugoslavia. By 1960, it was no longer permitted in Morocco, Turkey, or Uruguay, but was approved for use in Bulgaria and Thailand. It is believed to have been used in foods in Japan from 1948 until 1965, when approval was retained only for certain non-food uses (536).

This compound has been classified as a color found to be harmful, and which should not be used in food (438,537). The toxicological evidence on which this decision was based can be derived from an unpublished document (3) and reference 538.

More recently, the carcinogenic potential of this color has been examined and it was concluded that ponceau 3R is carcinogenic in rats following its oral administration, producing liver-cell tumors. It also produced bladder tumors in mice following its implantation in the urinary bladder. The oral study in mice, however, was considered inadequate for evaluation (539).

One review on the toxicology of this compound (540) and no review on its specifications is available. Some information is also found in reference 538.

PONCEAU 4R

This compound was classified in the category of food colors for which the available data were inadequate for evaluation, but for which a substantial amount of detailed information was available concerning results of long-term tests (438,541).

---

*This reference refers to this compound as ponceau MX.

In a subsequent evaluation, several long-term studies in the rat were examined and a temporary ADI for man of 0.75 mg/kg bw was established, based on a demonstrated no-effect level in studies in the rat (150 mg/kg bw/day). Metabolic studies in several animal species, preferably including man and a two-year study in a non-rodent mammalian species were requested (542,543).

In a further evaluation, additional long-term studies were examined; since the long-term study in mice indicated a no-effect level of 25 mg/kg bw/day, the temporary ADI for man was lowered at 0.125 mg/kg bw. It was observed that several long-term studies specifically designed for carcinogenesis had been performed in the rat, and one in the mouse; teratology has been examined in the mouse and a short-term study in a non-rodent species has been performed. It was, however, noted that little information on the metabolism was available (544,545). This ADI for man was subsequently extended (39).

Indicated areas for further research comprise metabolic studies in several animal species, preferably including man; and adequate long-term studies in another species; as well as reproduction studies (544, 546).

The Scientific Committee for Food of the Commission of the European Communities established a temporary ADI for man of 0.15 mg/kg bw for this color and requested the results of metabolic studies in animals and, if possible, in man, as well as of a long-term study in rats and a reproduction study (368).

Three reviews on the toxicology of this compound (547,548,549) and four reviews on its specifications (550,551,552,553) are available. Analytical aspects are found in references, 397, 554, and 555. Some information is also found in reference 556.

PONCEAU 6R

This monoazo compound was classified in the category of food colors for which the available data were inadequate for evaluation, and for which virtually no information on long-term toxicity was available. Colors with long-term tests for tumor formation, unaccompanied by other long-term studies, were considered as falling within this category (438, 557).

In subsequent evaluations, it was noted that no information on the metabolismoof this compound was available. The long-term studies performed were aimed solely at discovering potential carcinogenicity and, therefore, did not include the detailed observations usually made in these tests. Only small numbers of animals were used, so that these experiments were inadequate to assess long-term toxicity. Information on reproductive effects and embryotoxicity, including teratogenicity, was absent. Sensitization in man had been reported after oral intake. No ADI for man was established (545,558). Furthermore, no information was available that any manufacturer produces this color for food use (559).

Indicated areas for further research comprise adequate long-term studies in two animal species, as well as reproduction and embryotoxicity, including teratogenicity studies (558).

The Scientific Committee for Food of the Commission of the European Communities endorsed the opinion of not establishing an ADI for man because of the inadequacy of data, and it classified this color among food colors for which an ADI could not be established and which are not toxicologically acceptable for use in food (494).

One review on the toxicology of this compound (560) and two reviews on its specifications (561,562) are available. Analytical aspects are found in reference 397. Some information is also found in reference 563.

PONCEAU SX

The preparation of this monoazo compound was first reported in 1886. In 1972, in the U.S., this monoazo color was manufactured by two companies. In Western Europe, there may be as many as five producers of ponceau SX, but current production is believed to be small. It is not produced commercially in Japan at present.

It has been reported that ponceau SX was approved for food use in Australia, Canada, Greece, Japan, Mexico, the Netherlands, New Zealand, Norway, Peru, South Africa, the United Kingdom, and the U.S. A later report indicates additional approvals in Cuba, Denmark, the Dominican Republic, Finland, Guatemala, Israel, the Philippines, Sweden, and Uruguay; but indicates that approval had been withdrawn in The Netherlands. More recently, it has been reported that its use in foods has been approved in Austria. In Japan, ponceau SX was permitted in foodstuffs from 1948 until 1966, when it was approved only for certain nonfood uses.

In the U.S., it was on the list of food colors approved under the U.S. Pure Food and Drug Act of 1906 and it has been reported that ponceau SX was used as a coloring in the following products: gelatin desserts, maraschino cherries, frozen desserts, carbonated beverages, dry drink powders, confectionery products, spaghetti, puddings, aqueous drug solutions, tablets, capsules, ointments, bath salts, and hair rinses.

However, its general use in foods, drugs, and cosmetics has not been permitted since June 1965, because of adverse toxicological evidence. At present, it is only permitted in the U.S. for use in the coloring of maraschino cherries at a level not exceeding 150 mg/kg by weight of the cherries. It may be used in ingested drugs, provided that the labeling does not recommend or suggest continuous administration (maximum, six weeks) and that the amount of ponceau SX used is such that not more than 5 mg are consumed per day. It may be used in externally applied drugs and cosmetics without restriction. This color is now listed provisionally and its status reviewed every six months (564). In a subsequent evaluation, it was observed that apparently no manufacturer produces this color for food use.

This color has been classified as a color found to be harmful, and which should not be used in food (299). The toxicological evidence on which this decision was based is derived from reference 3 and partially from reference 565.

Limited metabolic data and adequate long-term studies were available in the rat and mouse. These studies indicated no carcinogenic effects at the higher level fed (5 percent). In the dog, there was a dose-related atrophy of the adrenal zona glomerulosa, as well as hemorrhagic lesions and blood-filled mucosal projections into the urinary bladder at all dose levels. An ADI for man could not be established until further studies in the dog were undertaken to define the no-effect level. In addition, a multi-generation reproduction/teratology study would also be required (566).

In an evaluation of the carcinogenic potential of this compound, it was noted that ponceau SX was tested by the oral route in mice, rats, and dogs, and by subcutaneous injections in mice and rats; no carcinogenic effect was observed in these experiments (567).

Two reviews on the toxicology of this compound (23,568) and one on its specifications (569) are available. Some information is also in reference 565.

QUERCITIN/QUERCITRON

Quercitron is obtained from the inner bark of Quercus tinctoria, a species of oak tree. The coloring principle is quercitin ($C_{21}H_{20}O_{11}$). It is one of the most important, as well as the most abundant, of the dyes of the flavone type. It is insoluble in water, but soluble in alkalis, giving it a yellow color (570).

These materials were classified in the category of food colors for which the available data were inadequate for evaluation, but for which a substantial amount of detailed information was available concerning results of long-term tests (438,571).

In a subsequent evaluation, it was noted that in a short-term study in rats, the animals developed cataracts within two weeks of stomach intubation. The same effect was not observed with the chromatographically pure compound, however, which led to the attributing of this effect to impurities contained in the commercial quercitin. No acceptable daily intake for man (ADI) was established.

Indicated areas for further research comprise information on the occurrence of toxic impurities in commercial samples of quercitin and quercitron, on the metabolic fate of these compounds, adequate long-term studies in a rodent species, and a two-year study in a non-rodent mammalian species (572,573).

In addition, it was observed that there was no evidence that any manufacturer produces these materials for food use. Subsequently, it was noted that quercitin demonstrated positive mutagenic effects in two strains of Salmonella typhimurium; however, the purity of the material tested was not reported (574).

Two reviews on the toxicology of these substances (573,575) and one review on its specifications (576) are available. Some information is also found in reference 570.

QUINOLINE YELLOW

Initially, this quinophthalone compound was classified in the category of colors for which the available data were inadequate for evaluation, and for which virtually no information on long-term toxicity was available (438). Subsequently, results of long-term studies provided justification for including this color in the category of food colors for which the available data were inadequate for evaluation, but for which is substantial amount of information was available concerning results of long-term tests (577,578).

In a further evaluation, a temporary ADI for man of 1 mg/kg bw was established for this color on a demonstrated no-effect level in the rat (50 mg/kg bw/day) (579,580). Metabolic studies in several animal species, preferably including man, and a two-year study in a non-rodent mammalian species were requested.

The compound was again examined subsequently and a temporary ADI for man of 0.5 mg/kg bw was allocated, based on the no-effect previously demonstrated in the rat (50 mg/kg bw/day), but using a smaller safety factor. Metabolic studies in several animal species, preferably including man; adequate long-term studies in another species; and multigeneration studies were requested (581,582). In a further evaluation, the temporary ADI for man of 0.5 mg/kg bw was retained (583,584) and it was observed that there were two commercial preparations of this food color; one of which contains about 30 percent of the methylated color; while the other contains only the non-methylated color. However, the specifications (585) covered both types of commercial products.

Since in the manufacture of these colors, the impurities are qualitatively the same, the toxicological data obtained on the color containing the methylated derivative could be used as collateral evidence to also ensure the safety of the non-methylated preparation. There is no biological information on either preparation; however, an adequate long-term study in rats is available. Additional studies on non-rodents have become available for evaluation; embryotoxicity and teratogenicity have already been studied in two animal species.

Indicated areas for further research included metabolic studies in several species, preferably including man; adequate long-term studies in other species; and multi-generation studies (586).

In a further evaluation, newly available teratogenicity studies in the rat and rabbit were examined. No adverse teratogenic effects were noted at dietary levels up to 150 mg/kg bw. In a three-generation reproduction study, in which quinoline yellow was fed to rats at levels up to 50 mg/kg bw, no adverse effects were noted. The previously established ADI was extended for another period of time (39).

The Scientific Committee for Food of the Commission of the European Communities noted that the impurities were qualitatively the same in the manufacture of the two commercial products. Therefore, toxicological data obtained on the color containing the methylated derivative could be used as collateral evidence to assure the safety of the non-methylated preparation; it endorsed the temporary ADI of 0.5 mg/kg bw (79).

Five reviews on the toxicology of this compound (40,587,588,589, 590) and four on its specifications (585,591,592,593) are available. Analytical aspects are found in reference 594. Some information is also found in reference 595.

RED 10B

This monoazo compound was classified in the category of food colors for which the available data were inadequate for evaluation, and for which virtually no information on long-term toxicity was available. Compounds with long-term tests for tumor formation, unaccompanied by other long-term studies, were considering as falling within this category (438,596). The evidence on which this decision was based has not been published in the form of a monograph; it can, however, be found in an unpublished document (597).

When rabbits were fed 0.5 g/kg bw of the color, the following metabolites could be identified in urine within 48 hours: p-aminophenol, and o-aminophenol. Rats were injected intravenously and the bile was collected for six hours and analyzed; the recovery of the color was at an average of 12 percent (5-20 percent) of the administered quantity.

Groups of 10 weanling albino rats equally divided as to sex, were fed diets containing 0, 0.25, 0.5, 1.0, 2.0, and 5 percent for 90 days. Animals fed diets containing 5 percent of the color showed lowered hemoglobin and hematocrit values. The organs affected were the liver, kidney, and spleen. Liver and kidney enlargement was observed in animals fed at the 1.0, 2.0, and 5.0 percent levels. Splenic enlargement occurred at all dosage levels. Growth inhibition occurred at the 0.25, 0.5, and 2.0 percent levels. References to these studies are found in Table III.

The Scientific Committee for Food of the Commission of the European Communities, in evaluating this compound, has observed that the structure of this azo dye is closely related to that of red 2G, which hydrolyzes slowly in acid solution to give red 10B. From the analytical point of view, therefore, all food containing red 2G could contain traces of red 10B. Significant quantities of this hydrolysis product are likely to be found in products of high acidity and subjected to high temperature during processing. This phenomenon is not unique to these two colors. Red 10B has also been put forward as a color in its own right.

Only scanty metabolic information is available on red 10B. Information on short- and long-term tests in rats and dogs, as well as skin painting studies, is available only as a summary prepared by the U.S. Food and Drug Administration.

These studies showed that red 10B belongs to the class of compounds causing hemolytic anemia and Heinz body formation. The results of the long-term studies were not available in full, and could not be examined by the Committee; but even from the summaries available they appeared inadequate in terms of numbers of animals used and design, when judged by modern standards. No reproduction studies were available, but the summary of the teratology studies appeared to show no adverse effects.

On the basis of the data available, it is not possible to recommend that red 10B be used to color food. In addition, red 2G should not be used under conditions in which significant hydrolysis to red 10B occurs (723).

No review on the toxicology of this compound but one on its specifications (598) is available. Some information is also found in reference 599.

RED 2G

This monoazo compound was classified in the category of food colors for which the available data were inadequate for evaluation, and for which virtually no information on long-term toxicity was available. Compounds with long-term tests for tumor formation, unaccompanied by other long-term studies, were considered as falling within this category (600,601).

In a subsequent evaluation, several studies were examined. Metabolic data demonstrated that major metabolites in the rat and rabbit included aminophenols and aniline. Both short- and long-term toxicity studies in rats and mice showed depression of erythropoiesis and the production of Heinz bodies. The lowest no-effect level was obtained in a short-term rat study when the color was incorporated into sausage meat comprising 80 percent of the diet. In this study, the no-effect level was about 25 ppm, in terms of the whole diet. On that basis, a temporary ADI for man was established at 0.006 mg/kg bw, and further work comprising a multigeneration reproduction/teratology study and studies on bone marrow to elucidate the toxic effects on erythropoiesis, were requested (602).

The Scientific Committee for Food of the Commission of the European Communities established an ADI of 0.1 mg/kg bw and classified this color in the category of food colors for which an ADI for man could be established, and which are, therefore, toxicologically acceptable for use in food within the ADI's limits (78).

One review on the toxicology of this compound (23) and two reviews on its specifications (603,604) are available. Analytical aspects are found in references 347 and 605. Some information is also found in reference 606.

RESORCINE BROWN

This disazo compound was classified in the category of food colors for which the available data were inadequate for evaluation, and for which virtually no information on long-term toxicity was available. Compounds with long-term tests for tumor formation, unaccompanied by other long-term studies, were considered as falling within the category (600,607). The evidence for this decision is partially found in an unpublished document (608).

Five groups of 20 rats each were fed the color for 90 days. Dosage levels were 0, 0.25, 0.5, 1.0, and 2.0 percent. No gross effects were observed. Reference to this study is found in Table III.

No review on the toxicology of this compound or on its specifications are available.

RHODAMINE B

This xanthene compound was classified in the category of food colors for which the available information was inadequate for evaluation, but indicated the possibility of harmful effects. It was reported as producing more than 10-15 percent of local sarcomas at the site of repeated subcutaneous injection (600,609). The toxicological evidence on which this decision was based is found in reference 610 and partially in reference 611.

In the U.S., this color is provisionally listed for use in drugs and cosmetics, subject to certification. Certified rhodamine B must meet the product specifications. Its use in drug products for internal use and in mouthwashes, dentifrices, and proprietary products is limited to a maximum tolerance level of 0.75 mg, the amount of product reasonably expected to be ingested in one day. In lipsticks, the maximum amount of all colors used, including rhodamine B, is limited to a maximum of 6 percent pure dye by weight of each lipstick. It may be used without tolerance levels in other externally applied cosmetics and drugs. In Western Europe, it may be used in cosmetics, including those which may be in contact with mucous membranes (612).

In an evaluation of the carcinogenic potential of this color, it was noted that rhodamine B has been tested in mice and rats by subcutaneous injection and, in inadequate studies, by oral administration. It was found to be carcinogenic in rats when injected subcutaneously, producing local sarcomas (613).

One review on the toxicology of this compound (614) and one on its specifications (615) are available. Some information is also found in reference 611. Analytical aspects are found in reference 397.

RHODAMINE 6G

This xanthene compound was classified in the category of food colors for which the available data were inadequate for evaluation, and for which virtually no information on long-term toxicity was available. Compounds with long-term tests for tumor formation, unaccompanied by other long-term studies, were considered as falling within this category. This compound produced more than 10-15 percent of local sarcomas at the site of repeated subcutaneous injection (600,607). The toxicoligical evidence for this decision is found in refer nce 616 and partially in reference 617.

In Western Europe, rhodamine 6G may provisionally be used in cosmetics which may come into contact with mucous membranes (618).

In the evaluation of the carcinogenic potential of this color, it was noted that rhodamine 6G was found to be carcinogenic in rats after its subcutaneous injection, producing sarcomas and that it has been inadequately tested in mice by oral administration (619).

One review on the toxicology of this compound (620) and no review on its specifications are available. Some information is also found in reference 617.

RIBOFLAVIN

Riboflavin is a yellow substance extracted from natural sources or manufactured synthetically; it contains no less than 98 percent and no more than 102 percent of $C_{17}H_{20}N_4O_6$, calculated on a dry basis. It is commercially available as a yellow to orange-yellow powder sparingly soluble in water (621).

In a previous evaluation, riboflavin was considered to be technologically unsuitable for use as a food color and it has been recommended that its use in food should be based upon its properties as a vitamin (622).

In a subsequent evaluation, based on a no-effect level in the rat (50 mg/kg bw/day) an acceptable daily intake for man of 0.5 mg/kg bw was established to this color for its use as a food additive. Animals fed high doses of riboflavin show no toxic effects. There are several biochemical studies and a vast amount of clinical and nutritional data on riboflavin; this information has been extensively used in its evaluation for use solely as a food additive (623,624).

The Scientific Committee for Food of the Commission of the European Communities was presented with information on riboflavin-5'-phosphate and additional data was considered. Since this compound is a normal metabolite of riboflavin, no objection was expressed as to the use of this substance to color food despite the absence of extensive animal toxicological data. However, the opinion was expressed that, because of the photo-chemical instability of this substance, the problem of breakdown products required investigation, and that the use of this substance to color food should not significantly alter the average daily intake of riboflavin. It was also recommended that riboflavin should be maintained on the list of permitted coloring matter. (722).

One review on the toxicology of this substance (625) and one review on its specifications (621) are available. Some information is also found in reference 626.

SAFFRON/CROCIN/CROCETIN

These carotenoid materials were not evaluated because the lack of toxicological information and the lack of knowledge of composition, the variation in composition according to the source, and the method of preparation employed (14). Furthermore, crocin and crocetin are not produced as food colors commercially (627).

Saffron is the dried powdered stigma of Crocus sativus L. It usually contains 4-6 percent of the main coloring principles; crocin and crocetin. Saffron is a red-brown or golden-yellow odoriferous powder; it has a slightly bitter taste, and distinct odor (628). Crocin is a water-soluble orange-red carotenoid.

Saffron, with or without approved diluent, may be used under the U.S. Federal Food, Drug, and Cosmetic Act concerning coloring of foods, without a requirement for certification. It is also allowed in Canada as a food additive that may be used as a coloring agent at levels of use consistent with good manufacturing practice. Saffron has been widely used as carminative, diaphoretic, and even abortient. It should be noted that prostaglandins also chemically resemble α-crocin.

A 28-year old female ingested 20 tablets of Cyren-B and about 5 g of saffron to induce an abortion. Serious reactions developed temporarily, including localized skin hemorrhages, caused by severe histologically demonstrated damage to capillaries and precapillaries, thrombocytopenia, and abnormalities of blood clotting.

Oral LD_{50} of a decoction of Crocus sativus in mice was 20.7 g (crude drug)/kg. Mice fed diets containing 0.23-2 percent of Crocus sativus L. powder for three weeks showed the duration of complete cornification of vaginal epithelium prolonged from the normal 1-2 days to 3-4 days. References to these studies are found in Table III. No acceptable daily intake for man was established for these materials (627).

No review on the toxicology of these materials but two reviews are available on the specifications of saffron (628,629). Analytical aspects are found in reference 628. Some information is also found in reference 630.

SCARLET GN

This monoazo compound was classified in the category of food colors for which the available data were inadequate for evaluation, and for which virtually no information on long-term toxicity was available. Compounds with long-term tests for tumor formation, unaccompanied by other long-term studies, were considered as falling within this category (600, 631). The toxicological evidence for this decision is found in reference 632 and partially in reference 633.

It appears that no source or use of scarlet GN as a food color can be found. Studies available consist of limited mutagenic and short-term toxicity studies, as well as a long-term study in the rat. However, the number of animal studies was insufficient, and there was a lack of detail regarding the factors measured. No acceptable daily intake for man was established for this compound (634).

Groups of rats were intravenously injected with scarlet GN (an amount molecularily equivalent to 1 mg of 4-dimethylaminoazobenzene per kg) and the percentage of coloring excreted in the bile after six hours was measured spectrophotometrically. No detectable amount of scarlet GN was recovered in the bile. This color was tested for mutagenic effect in a concentration of 0.5 g/100 ml in cultures of Escherichia coli. No mutagenic effect was found.

Five rats were orally given 1.5 g/kg bw for 22 days. No Heinz bodies were found. In experiments with guinea-pigs, it was found that this color had no sensitization activity. A negative test for Heinz bodies was found when two cats were given per os 0.1 g/kg bw for seven days.

The oral LD_{50} in the mouse is of the order of >5 g/kg bw; the intravenous in the rat is in the range of 1-2.5 g/kg bw and the intraperitoneal of >2 g/kg bw.

Ten rats were given 1 percent of the color in their drinking water for 233 days. The average daily intake was 0.98 g per kg bw and the total intake was 50 g/animal. The observation period was 575 days. No tumors were found.

Twelve rats were given a diet containing 1 percent of the color in their drinking water for 248 days. The average daily intake was 1.2 g/kg bw; the total intake was 50 g/animal. The animals were kept under observation for 880 days. No tumors were noted. Five rats died before the end of the experiment.

Ten rats were fed the color at a level of 0.1 percent in the diet for 410 days. The average daily dose was 0.06 g/kg bw; the total intake 6g/animal. The animals were kept under observation for 761 days. No tumors were observed.

Ten rats were given subcutaneous injections twice weekly for 52 weeks, of 0.5 ml of a 1 percent solution. Total amount applied was 0.5 g/animal. The animals were kept under observation for 1,180 days. One polymorphocellular sarcoma was found in the liver. References to these studies are found in Table III.

The Scientific Committee for Food of the Commission of the European Communities endorsed the decision of not establishing an ADI for man for this compound, and it classified this color among those food colors for which an ADI could not be established, and which are not toxicologically acceptable for use in food (494).

No review on the toxicology of this compound, but two reviews on its specifications (636) are available. Analytical aspects are found in reference 397. Some information is also found in reference 633.

SILVER

Silver as a food coloring agent was considered, but no attempt was made at a toxicological evaluation (600,607).

Silver toxicity is manifested in man in a variety of forms, some proven others suspected. Proven forms include: argyria, gastrointestinal irritation, and renal and pulmonary lesions. Suspected forms include, among others (ill-defined) arteriosclerosis.

Argyria denotes the slate blue color observed in parts of the body of persons chronically exposed to silver. Epidemiologically, two types of argyria are recognized: industrial argyria and iatrogenic argyria.

Regardless of type, there are two forms of argyria: local and generalized. The local form involves the formation of grey blue patches on the skin, or may manifest itself in the conjuctiva of the eye. In generalized argyria, the skin shows widespread pigmentation, often spreading from the face to most uncovered parts of the body. In some cases, the skin may become black with a metallic luster. Heavy pigmentation of the dye structures can interfere with vision. Except for this adverse effect, argyria is solely a cosmetic problem. The slate blue color of argyria is not entirely due, as one might suspect, to the deposition of metallic silver, but largely to an increased deposition of melanin. Silver has a melanocyte-stimulating property. Cases of generalized argyria have occurred after ingestion or chronic medicinal application of gram quantities of silver. Silver was absorbed during prolonged (nine months) nasal application of Targesine (silver solution). It was calculated that during this time 7,000 ml of solution, containing 210 g silver, had been used.

The systemic effects of silver are not extensive because of the poor absorption of silver compounds from the intestinal tract. It is considered that 10 g of silver nitrate taken orally is a lethal dose for man, although recovery from smaller doses has been reported. The systemic effects of a lethal dose are preceded by severe hemorrhagic gastroenteritis and shock. The silver ion seems first to stimulate and then depress structures in the brain stem. Central vasomotor stimulation results in a rise in blood pressure. At the same time, there is bradycardia due to central vagal stimulation. Death eventually results from respiratory depression. References to these studies are found in Table III.

This metal is rarely used in food; the exact nature of silver used on or in food is not known. The data available suggest that silver might accumulate in certain tissues following long-term exposure. The data, however, are insufficient to evaluate this point fully, and no adequate long-term feeding studies are available. Consequently, no acceptable daily intake for man has been established (637).

Because of the inadequacy of the available biological information on silver, the Scientific Committee for Food of the Commission of the European Communities concluded that an ADI for man could not be established; however, the use of silver for surface coloring and decoration of food has been accepted without further investigation (77).

One review on the toxicology of this substance as a food color (23) is available, but there are no specifications.

SUDAN I

This monoazo compound has been classified as a color found to be harmful, and which should not be used in food (600,639). The toxicological evidence on which this decision was made can be derived from reference 3 and partially from reference 638.

Sudan I was first prepared in 1883. In 1972, six U.S. manufacturers reported production of about 270,000 kg. In Western Europe, there may be as many as 16 producers of sudan I, with a total current production estimated at 100,000 kg per year. In Japan in 1972, six manufacturers reported production of 46,000 kg of this color.

It has been reported that this compound was approved for use in food coloring in Belgium, Egypt, Italy, Norway, Poland, Portugal, Rumania, South Africa, Switzerland, and Turkey. A later report indicated that such approval had subsequently been withdrawn in Belgium, Norway, Portugal, and South Africa (640).

In a recent evaluation of the carcinogenic potential of this compound, it was observed that sudan I is carcinogenic in mice following its subcutaneous administration, producing tumors of the liver. It also produced bladder tumors in mice following its implantation into the urinary bladder. Tests by oral administration in mice and rats were negative, but the adequacy of the dose level used could not be assessed (641).

One review on the toxicology of this compound (642), and no review on its specifications are available. Some information is also found in reference 638.

SUDAN III

This disazo compound has been classified in the category of colors for which the available data are inadequate for evaluation, and for which virtually no information on long-term toxicity is available. Compounds with long-term tests for tumor formation, unaccompanied by other long-term studies, were considered as falling within this category (600, 643). The toxicological evidence on which this decision was based has not been published but it can be derived from reference 3 and partially from reference 644.

Sudan III was first prepared in 1879. In 1972, only one U.S. manufacturer reported production. There may be as many as 14 producers of sudan III in Western Europe, but production is believed to be small. In Japan, four producers manufactured 3,400 kg of this color in 1972.

It has been reported that sudan III was approved for general food use in the USSR prior to 1955, but approval had been withdrawn by 1957.

In the U.S., on December 31, 1968, sudan III and all mixtures containing it were disallowed for use in ingested products; at present, it is permitted for use in certain non-food applications, at least in the U.S. and Japan (645).

In a recent evaluation of the carcinogenic potential of this compound, it was observed that it was administered to mice and rats by the oral route, and to mice by the subcutaneous route, but all experiments were inadequate for evaluation with regard to either the dose administered, the degree of reporting, and/or the number of animals used (646). References to these studies are found in Table III.

One review on the toxicology of this compound (647) and no review on its specifications is available. Some information is also found in reference 644.

SUDAN IV

This disazo compound has been classified in the category of food colors for which the available data were inadequate for evaluation, but indicated the possibility of harmful effects (600,643). The toxicological evidence on which this decision was based can be derived from reference 648 and partially from reference 649. References to these studies are found in Table III.

Sudan IV was synthesized in 1887. In 1972, there were three manufacturers of this color in the U.S. In Western Europe, there may be as many as 17 manufacturers of this substance, but it is believed that production is small. In Japan, seven producers manufactured 41,000 kg of sudan IV in 1972.

This color has reportedly been found to be useful in veterinary and human medicine as a four to eight percent of ointment for stimulating wound healing; dressings containing sudan IV and allantoin have been used in the management of indolent ulcers; and a 5 percent suspension in castor oil containing 1 percent atropine has been used in the treatment of corneal ulcers.

In Japan, sudan IV has approval for certain non-food usages and is believed to be used in paint colorants, printing inks, plastics, gasoline, petroleum products, cosmetics, and drugs applied externally (except on lips and mucous membranes).

It has been reported that the compound was approved in France for use in food coloring (e.g. of cheese rinds) prior to 1955; a later report indicated that this approval had been withdrawn (650).

In a recent evaluation of the carcinogenic potential of sudan IV, it was observed that the color induced local sarcomas in rats, following its subcutaneous injection; another experiment in which mice were treated orally gave negative results, but the adequacy of the dose could not be assessed. Other experiments were considered inadequate for evaluation (651).*

One review on the toxicology of this compound (652) and no review on its specifications is available. Some information is also found in reference 649.

SUDAN G

This monoazo compound has been classified in the category of food colors for which the available information was inadequate for evaluation,

---

*This reference reports this compound as scarlet red.

and for which virtually no information on long-term toxicity was available. Colors with long-term tests for tumor formation, unaccompanied by other long-term studies, were considered as falling within this category (600,643). The toxicological evidence on which this decision was based is derived from reference 653 and partially from reference 654.

The oral LD_{50} in the mouse is approximately 5 g/kg bw and the intraperitoneal LD_{50} in the rat in the order of 0.6 g/kg bw. Eighty-five rats were ed this color at a level of 0.1 percent in the diet. Each animal ingested 10-15 mg per day. No tumors were observed.

Groups of 20 and 10 rats equally divided by sex were given one and five percent of the color in the diet, respectively. All the animals refused the diet and the experiment was stopped.

Another experiment was with 15 male and 15 female rats that were given 0.5 percent of the color for 90 days; as control, 20 rats were used. During the experiment, two rats from the experimental group died. At the end of the experiment, no abnormalities were found in the blood picture. The composition of the urine did not show abnormalities. The growth of the test animals was decreased; but the weight of the spleen was incresed. In the liver, kidney, and spleen; an endogenous pigment was deposited.

A positive test for Heinz bodies was obtained after feeding a cat 0.1 g/kg bw of this color for seven days, and another cat 0.002 g/kg bw for 33 days.

A total of 137 male and female mice produced by mixed breeding from five different strains was given a diet containing 2 mg per animal per day of the color. Mice at the age of 50 to 100 days were used. A number of the animals was sacrificed after an observation period of 500 days, and the rest of the survivors after 700 days. A total of 168 mice was used as negative controls. Positive control groups which were given o-aminoazotoluene and dimethylaminoazobenzene, were also included. In these groups the formation of liver tumors was noted after approximately 200 days. The incidence of tumors in mice receiving the color was not significantly greater than in the negative controls.

Eighty-nine rats were fed 9 mg per day for periods up to 900 days. The total intake of the color was 7.5 g per animal. No tumors were observed. References to these studies were found in Table III.

No review on the toxicology of this compound but one review on its specifications (655) is available. Some information is also found in reference 654.

SUDAN RED G

This monoazo compound has been classified in the category of food colors for which the available data were inadequate for evaluation, and for which virtually no infor ation on long-term toxicity was available. Compounds with long-term tests for tumor formation, unaccompanied by other long-term studies, were considered as falling within this category (600,656). The toxicological evidence on which this decision was based is derived from reference 657 and partially from reference 658.

The oral LD_{50} in the mouse is of the order of 3 g/kg bw. Two groups of twenty rats, 10 males and 10 females, were given none and one percent; and 10 rats, five percent of the color in the diet for 90 days. In the group with five percent, a clear decrease in growth was found. At the end of the experiment, no abnormalities were found in the blood pictures. The composition of the urine did not show abnormalities. In the spleen and kidney, pigment deposits were found. The organ weights were not measured.

A cat was given 0.1 g/kg bw of this color per day for seven days. A positive test for Heinz bodies was obtained. Similar results were observed with a cat fed 0.002 g/kg bw for 33 days.

One hundred and twenty-seven rats were fed 8 mg of this color daily, until a total of 6.6 g per animal had been ingested. The animals were kept under observation for 850 days. No tumors were observed. References to these studies are found in Table III.

No review on the toxicology of this compound but one on its specifications (659) is available. Some information is also found in reference 658.

SUNSET YELLOW FCF

This monoazo compound appears to have been first prepared in 1878. In 1972, six U.S. manufacturers reported a total production of 369,000 kg. In Western Europe, there are believed to be 15 manufacturers of sunset yellow FCF, with a total annual production estimated at several hundred thousand kg. In Japan, in 1973, seven producers manufactured about 203,000 kg; about 22,000 were exported in 1972 and 8,000 kg in 1973.

It has been reported that this material was approved for use as a general food coloring in Australia, Austria, Canada, the Federal Republic of Germany, Greece, Italy, Japan, Mexico, New Zealand, the Netherlands, Norway, Peru, South Africa, Spain, Sweden, Switzerland, the United Kingdom, the U.S., and Yugoslavia. A later report indicates additional approvals in Cuba, Denmark, the Dominican Republic, Egypt, Finland, Guatemala, India, Israel, the Philippines, and Uruguay; but indicated that approval had been withdrawn in Italy and Switzerland.

A recent report indicated that sunset yellow FCF was permitted for food, drug, and cosmetic use in a number of EEC countries; according to another source, all Western European countries except Portugal currently permit the use of this color in foods. It has been estimated that 95 percent of the sunset yellow FCF consumed in Japan is in food; and the remainder is in drugs, cosmetics, and inks.

Sunset yellow FCF is being used in gelatin, frozen desserts, carbonated beverages, dry drink powders, confectionary products, bakery products, cereals, puddings, aqueous drug solutions, tablets, capsules, toothpaste, and hair rinses. A U.S. consumption pattern for this color in foods, drugs, and cosmetics for the first nine months of 1967 was reported as follows: sweets and confections, 24,000 kg/ beverages, 82,400 kg; dessert powders, 23,500 kg; cereals, 16,100 kg; maraschino cherries, 2,200 kg; pet food, 10,500 kg; bakery goods, 19,100 kg; ice cream, sherbet, and dairy products, 10,300 kg; sausages, 45,300 kg; snack foods 5,200 kg; and miscellaneous, 13,200 kg; for a total consumption in food of about 250,000 kg. Pharmaceutical consumption was reported to be about 7,250 kg and cosmetic consumption about 1,000 kg. The maximum quantity of this color ingested in the U.S. per capita, per day, per food category during this period was estimated to be as follows: sweets and confections, 1.8 mg; beverages, 4.1 mg; dessert powders, 1.8 mg; cereals, 0.5 mg; maraschino cherries, 0.06 mg; bakery goods, 3.6 mg; ice cream, sherbet and dairy products, 1.3 mg; sausages, 1.8 mg; snack foods, 0.3 mg; and miscellaneous, 0.2 mg (660).

Several long-term studies have been carried out in mice, rats, and dogs. The biochemical studies indicate that in the rat, this color is reduced at the azo linkage by bacteria present in the intestine and that some of the breakdown products are absorbed and then excreted in the urine.

No-effect levels have been demonstrated in the rat at five percent (50,000 ppm) and in the dog at two percent (20,000 ppm) in the diet (equivalent to 500 mg/kg bw/day) and an estimate of ADI for man of 5 mg/kg bw was established based on the long-term studies in dogs (661, 662).

Indicated areas for further desirable research on this compound comprise metabolic studies and reproduction studies in several animal species and research on the combined effect with amaranth and tartrazine (661).

In a recent evaluation of the carcinogenic potential of this compound, it was observed that experimental studies were carried out on this color in mice and rats by the oral route, and in rats by the subcutaneous route. In the oral experiments in mice, there was no evidence of carcinogenicity as compared with controls. Tests in rats by the oral route showed negative results; but the experiments were inadequately reported. Repeated subcutaneous injections in rats led to neither local nor distant tumors (663).

The Scientific Committee for Food of the Commission of the European Communities classified this color among the food colors for which an acceptable daily intake for man could be established, and which is, therefore, toxicologically acceptable for use in food within the ADI's limits. It established an ADI of 2.5 mg/kg bw for this compound considering new available information (78).

Two reviews on the toxicology of this compound (664,665) and two on its specifications (665,666) are available. Analytical aspects are found in reference 397. Some information is also found in reference 667.

TARTRAZINE

Several long-term studies have been carried out on this monoazo compound in the rat. Results from biochemical and metabolic studies show that tartrazine can be reduced in vivo in the rat, when given orally, but not intraperitoneally, to the rat. The reduction is therefore carried out by the gastrointestinal flora. This finding seems to indicate the possible absence of a true azo-linkage, and it was demonstrated by physical methods that tartrazine was the ketohydrazone tautomer. Cleavage of this tautomer by the flora of the gastrointestinal tract appears to have its counterpart in man, because experiments revealed no unchanged color in the urine. Biochemical studies with this color in the rat and rabbit are fairly extensive. A no-effect level has been demonstrated in the rat (750 mg/kg bw/day) and this served as a basis for estimating an ADI for man of 7.5 mg/kg bw (668,669).

Indicated areas for further desirable research comprise metabolic studies in more animal species, reproduction studies in several animal species, and research on the combined effect with amaranth and sunset yellow FCF (670).

The Scientific Committee for Food of the Commission of the European Communities classified this color among the food colors for which an acceptable daily intake for man could be established, and which are, therefore, toxicologically acceptable for use within the ADI's limit. In endorsing the figure of 7.5 mg/kg bw, it was observed that hypersensitivity reactions have been reported in certain individuals ingesting this food color (78).

One review on the toxicology of this compound (671) and two on its specifications (671,672) are available. Analytical aspects are found in reference 397. Some information is also found in reference 673.

THIAZINE BROWN R

This disazo compound was classified in the category of food colors for which the available data were inadequate for evaluation, and for which virtually no information on long-term toxicity was available. Compounds with long-term tests for tumor formation, unaccompanied by other long-term studies, were considered as falling within this category. This compound produced more than 10-15 percent of local sarcomas at the site of repeated subcutaneous injection (600,643). The toxicological evidence for this decision is found in reference 674 and partially in reference 675.

The oral LD_{50} in the mouse is in the range of 1 g/kg bw; the intraperitoneal and intravenous LD_{50} in the rat are respectively in the order of 0.7 g and 0.25 g/kg bw.

This color was fed to four cats as a five percent aqueous solution in an amount of 1.0 g on the first day and 0.1 g on both the eighth and 19th day. A negative test for Heinz bodies was obtained.

Ten rats were fed a diet containing 0.1 percent of this color in an amount of 0.06 g/kg/bw per day, until the animals had ingested 10 g in 692 days. The animals were kept under observation for periods up to 884 days. No tumors were noted.

Ten rats were given subcutaneous injections of 0.5 ml of a 0.5 percent solution twice weekly for a period of 270 days, and were then kept under observation for periods up to 634 days. Sarcomas developed at the site of the injections in nine out of ten of the experimental animals. References to these studies are found in Table III.

No review on the toxicology or specification of this compound is available. Some information is also found in reference 675.

TITANIUM DIOXIDE

This inorganic compound has been classified in the category of food colorants for which the available data were inadequate for evaluation, but for which a substantial amount of detailed information was available concerning results of long-term tests (600,676).

Titanium dioxide is a very soluble compound. The studies in several species, including man, show neither significant absorption nor tissue storage following ingestion of titanium dioxide. Studies on soluble titanium compound have, therefore, not been reviewed. It is useful to note that following absorption of small amounts of titanium ions, no toxic effects were observed.

An ADI not specified* was allocated to this compound, since the evidence indicates that it is free from toxic effects because of its insolubility and inertness (677,678).

The Scientific Committee for Food of the Commission of the European Communities classified this compound in the category of food colorants for which an ADI for man could not be established, but which are nevertheless acceptable for external and/or mass coloring of sugar confectionery, without the need for further investigation (77). However, in a subsequent assessment, and considering new information on other potential uses and on specifications, the inclusion of this color in the list of colors for food use in general was recommended (724).

Two reviews on the toxicology of this compound (679,680) and two on its specifications (681,682) are available. Analytical aspects are found in references 683 and 681.

---

*See footnote on page 26.

TURMERIC/CURCUMIN

Turmeric consists of the ground rhizome Curcuma and Curcuma longa
V. which contains curcumin, an orange-yellow color as the main coloring principle. It usually contains 1-5 percent of curcumin. The color
appears as a yellow-brown powder, with characteristic flavor and taste.
It contains yellow gelatinized starch masses, vascular bundles, and
broken pieces of oil cells; it does not contain stone cells, collen-
chymatous cells, and raphids or rosette aggregates of calcium oxalate,
and should be free from a musty odor (684).

Curcumin is an orange-yellow, crystalline powder, insoluble in
water and ether, but soluble in ethanol and glucial acetic acid. In the
commercial product used for coloring food, the content of curcumin is
usually stated (685).

In a previous examination of these substances, no attempt at a
toxicological evaluation was made, because of the lack of toxicological
information and the lack of knowledge of composition, the variation in
composition according to the course, and the method of preparation employed (600,643).

Subsequently, a temporary ADI for man of 0.5 mg/kg bw was
allocated, only to turmeric. This figure was based on a no-effect level
demonstrated in a long-term study in the rat (250 mg/kg bw/day) (686,
687). The biological data on turmeric, however, were far from complete
and none was available for the isolated coloring principle, the diphen-
olic compound, curcumin (688).

These natural coloring matters were again examined subsequently and
a temporary ADI for man of 2.5 mg/kg bw was allocated to turmeric, and
0.1 mg/kg bw to curcumin, which was considered to be present in turmeric,
at a three-percent level (689,690).

No adverse effects in animal tests have been obtained with a turmeric preparation of undefined curcumin content at the only level tested.
The true no-effect level may well have been higher than the level chosen (691).

In a further evaluation, data were available from several in vitro
studies, showing that extracts of turmeric caused chromosome damage.
This information reinforced the need for the previously required studies
(690,692). Since there was information indicating that these long-term
feeding studies and a multigeneration study were in progress, the previously established ADI's for turmeric and for curcumin were extended
(39).

The Scientific Committee for Food of the Commission of the European
Communities did not establish an ADI for man for turmeric, because this
material is excluded from the provisions of the Community Directive on
food colors. It did not establish an ADI for man for curcumin, but felt
able to accept the use of this color for use in food generally, without
the need for further investigation. However, metabolic studies in several species and, if possible, in man; adequate long-term studies in
another animal species; and reproduction and embryotoxicity, including
teratogenicity studies, will be needed if considerable extension of use
of this color in food is contemplated at some future date (79).

Three reviews on the toxicology of these substances (40,687,690)
and three reviews on their specifications (684,693,694) are available.
Information on analytical aspects for turmeric is found in references
695 and 696; and for curcumin in reference 697. Some information is
also found in reference 698.

ULTRAMARINES

These inorganic coloring compounds are insoluble in water but
readily decomposed by acids with liberation of hydrogen sulfide. They
are obtained by grinding the mineral lapis lazuli, or are made by fusing
together kaolin, sodium carbonate (or sodium sulfate), sulfur, and carbon. They are blue, violet, red or green lumps of powder, insoluble in
water.

Ultramarine consists essentially of a rigid alumino-silicate framework in which anions and cations are held, which are to some extent
mobile. The cations are normally sodium ions; the anions sulphide and
polysulphide ions, together with some free radical sulphur. The rigid
framework is composed of SiO_4 tetrahedra with shared corners, in which
silicon ions are randomly replaced by aluminium ions in four-fold co-
ordination (699).

In a previous assessment of these coloring substances, no attempt
was made at a toxicological evaluation, because of the lack of toxicological information and the lack of knowledge of composition, the
variation in composition according to the source, and the methods of
preparation employed (600,643). In addition, no evidence was available
that these substances are found in food commodities moving in international trade (700). The available toxicity data, consisting of several
short-term rat studies and a teratology study, could not be related to
the specifications of these substances; hence, no evaluation could be
made (700). References to available toxicological studies are found in
Table III.

The Scientific Committee for Food of the Commission of the European
Communities noted that ultramarine is a polysulphide of sodium (or potassium lithium, or silver) alumino silicate of unknown constitution,
which is obtained by grinding mineral lapis lazuli or by fusing together
kaolin, sodium carbonate (or sulphate), sulphur, and carbon.

No information was available on the metabolism of this color. The
short-term study in rats established a no-effect level, but no other
animal data were available. It was not possible to recommend that ultramarine be used to color food (724).

One review on the toxicology of these compounds (23) and one on
their specifications (699) are available; analytical aspects are also
found in the latter reference.

VIOLAMINE R

This xanthene compound has been classified in the category of colors
for which the available data were inadequate for evaluation, and for
which virtually no information on long-term toxicity was available.
Compounds with long-term tests for tumor formation, unaccompanied by
other long-term studies, were considered as falling within this category
(600,643). The evidence for this decision is partially derived from an
unpublished document (701).

No biochemical, acute toxicity, or short-term and special studies
are available for this compound, whose use is mostly as a biological
stain. The available study is a carcinogenicity study in the rat.

Twenty rats were injected subcutaneously once a week for four
months. After this period, the injections were given once or twice
monthly for 506 days. The color was given as 1 ml of three percent
aqueous solution. Ten rats survived 300 days or more. Only in one of
the animals a tumor developed at the site of injection. This animal died
after 346 days. In six animals, hypertrophy of thymus was found. Refer-

ence to this study is found in Table III.

No review on the toxicology or specification of this compound is available.

VIOLET 5 BN*

This triarylmethane compound has been classified in the category of colorssfor which the available data were inadequate for evaluation, and for which virtually no information on long-term toxicity is available. Compounds with long tests for tumor formation, unaccompanied by other long-term studies, were considered as falling within this category (600,643). The evidence for this decision is partially derived from an unpublished document (702).

No biochemical, acute toxicity, or short-term and special studies are available for this compound, whose use is mostly as a biological stain.

The only available study is represented by a chronic study in the mouse. One case of leukemia, out of 10 female mice of the A2G strain, was found when the color was painted on the skin. The duration of the experiment was not defined. The other animals received the color in their drinking water. A total of one out of 70 treated animals has no statistical significance. Reference to this study is found in Table III.

No review on the toxicology of this compound and one on its specifications (703) are available. Some information is also found in reference 704.

WATER BLUE I

This triarylmethane compound has been classified in the category of colors for which the available data were inadequate for evaluation, and for which virtually no information on long-term toxicity is available. Compounds with long tests for tumor formation, unaccompanied by other long-term studies, were considered as falling within this category (600, 643). The evidence for this decision is partially derived from an unpublished document (705).

The only available study is represented by a short-term study in the rat. Two groups of 20 rats and one group of 10 rats, half males and half females, were given 0.0 and 10,000 ppm and 50,000 ppm respectively in their diet for 90 days. Growth, blood, and urine composition were normal. No histologic abnormalities were found in heart, lung, liver, kidney, and spleen of the animals, which were sacrificed five and 15 days after the administration of the color was stopped. Reference to this study is found in Table III.

No review on the toxicology of this compound or on its specifications is available. Some information is found in reference 706.

XANTHOPHYLLS

Xanthophylls are the yellow principle of green leaves and represent about 10 percent of the total coloring matter of commercial technical chlorophyll. They are obtained as yellow prisms with a metallic luster when crystallized from alcohols; they are soluble in fat and fat solvents and almost insoluble in petroleum ether (707).

---

*This name is also used for benzyl violet 4B (704).

They are considered as belonging to the class of carotenoids. Products available have so far been used chiefly as animal (poultry) feed additives to enhance the color of egg yolks and chicken fat. Two dry types are available: citranaxanthin (see profile for this compound on page 35). Synthesized from beta-apo-8'-carotenal in reaction with acetone; and dried tagetes meal, ground flower petals of Aztec marigold (Tagetes erecta L.) or dried algae (genus Spongioccum) (708).

No attempt was made, in a previous assessment of these substances, at a toxicological evaluation, because of the lack of toxicological information, and the lack of knowledge of composition, the variation in composition to the source, and the methods of preparation employed (600, 643,708).

The Scientific Committee for Food of the Commission of the European Communities could not establish an ADI for man, because no specific biological data were available; nevertheless, it recommended that xanthophylls prepared from natural foods by physical processes be accepted for use as a coloring matter in food without further investigation. It further suggested that the acceptable natural xanthophylls be defined as including the 3-hydroxy- and 3,3'-dihydroxy-derivatives of α-carotene, their naturally occurring mono- and di-epoxides, neoxanthin, neochrome, and the fatty acid esters of these compounds present in natural foods. Xanthophylls, therefore, have been classified in the category of food colors for which an ADI could not be established, but which are nevertheless acceptable for use in food generally (77).

In addition, the same committee was presented with a request to consider a xanthophyll which occurs naturally in flowers, including the Aztec Marigold. This product is antheraxanthin (5,6-epoxy-5,6-dihydro-beta,beta-carotene-3,3'-diol). The product intended for use as a food colorant is a hexane extract of the flower petals. It contains antheraxanthin at a level of about 30 percent in the form of a dipalmitate. No toxicological information was supplied, either on the xanthophylls or on the commercial oleoresin intended to be used as a food colorant. It was, therefore, recommended that antheraxanthin should not be used to color food (723).

No review on the toxicology of these compounds and one on their specifications (709) are available.

YELLOW 2G

This monoazo compound has been classified in the category of food colors for which virtually no toxicological data were available (600, 643). In a subsequent examination no attempt was made at a toxicological evaluation for the same reason (710).

When several toxicological studies became available, the compound was re-examined. Short-term studies in the rat and pig did not reveal any serious adverse toxic effect. Two long-term studies in the mouse and rat have been done, but the results were not completely reported. However, multigeneration, embryotoxicity, including teratological studies, were not available and information on metabolism was not adequate. Consequently, no ADI for man was established (711, 712).

Subsequently, results on long-term studies in mice and rats became available. A histopathological finding was the occurrence of lymphomas in mice treated with this compound. In the rat, a treatment-related decrease in renal concentrating ability was noted. The no-effect level for this response was 100 mg/kg bw and, on the basis of this study, a temporary ADI for man of 0.025 mg/kg bw was established. Further work required comprises reproduction/teratology studies, and metabolic studies in several animal species, preferably including man (713).

The Scientific Committee for Food of the Commission of the European Communities noted that the short-term studies in the rat and pig did not reveal any serious adverse toxicity, but the long-term study in rats demonstrated some questionable adverse effects on renal function and kidney weight, in one sex only, at the highest levels tested. The long-term study in mice showed considerable scatter in the incidence of lymphosarcomas in the different animal groups, compared with the incidence in contemporary and historical controls. For these reasons, the Committee established a temporary ADI for man of 0.01 mg/kg bw and requested submission of the results of multigeneration (including embryotoxicity and teratology) studies, as well as repetition of the long-term mouse study, with special emphasis on the assessment and review of the variability in incidence of lymphosarcomas in the strain of mouse used (79).

Two reviews on the toxicology of this compound (23,714) and one review on its specifications (715) are available. Information on analytical aspects are found in reference 716. Some information is also found in reference 717.

YELLOW 27175 N

Yellow 27175 N "especially pure," a monoazo compound, was classified in the category of food colors for which the available data were inadequate for evaluation, and for which virtually no information on long-term toxicity was available. Compounds with long-term tests for tumor formation, unaccompanied by other long-term studies, were considered as falling within this category (600,718). The toxicological evidence for this decision is partially derived from an unpublished document (719) and from reference 720.

The mouse oral LD_{50} was found to be in the range of 5 g/kg bw and the rat intraperitoneal and intravenous, in the range of 2 g/kg and 1.0-2.5 g/kg bw respectively.

Five rats were given 1.5 g/kg bw for 22 days. No Heinz bodies were found. In experiments with guinea-pigs it was found that this color had no sensitization activity. A negative test for Heinz bodies was obtained on a cat fed at a level of 0.1 g/kg bw/day for 7 days.

In their drinking water, ten rats were given 0.5 percent of the color for 446 days. The daily intake was 0.43 g per kg bw; the total intake was 50 g/animal; the observation period was 546 days. No tumors were found.

In their drinking water, ten rats were given 0.5 percent of the color for 447 days. The daily intake was 0.45 g/kg bw; the total intake was 50 g per animal; the observation period was 891 days. In two animals, tumors of different types were found.

Ten rats were fed this color at a level of 0.1 percent in the diet for 410 days. The average daily dose was 0.06 g/kg bw. The animals were kept under observation for periods up to 761 days. One animal died before the end of the experiment, but no tumors were observed.

Ten rats were given subcutaneous injections twice weekly of 0.5 ml of a 1 percent solution of this color for 365 days, at which time a total of 0.5 g per animal had been injected. The animals were kept under observation for 895 days. No tumors developed.

No review on the toxicology of this compound and one on its specifications (718) are available. Some information is also found in reference 720.

REFERENCES

1. WHO/FAO. Specifications for the identity and purity of food additives and their toxicological evaluation: food colours and some antimicrobials and antioxidants. Eighth report. FAO Nutrition Meetings Report Series, No. 38; Wld. Hlth. Org. Techn. Rep. Ser., No. 309, 1965, p. 21.
2. WHO. Data sheets on food colours. WHO/Food Add./I Rev. 1, 1957, p. 120.
3. WHO. Monographs on food colours. Unpublished WHO document resulting from the eighth meeting of the Joint FAO/WHO Expert Committee on Food Additives in 1964, 1966, p. 2.
4. WHO. Specifications for identity and purity and toxicological evaluation of food colours. FAO Nutrition Meetings Report Series, No. 38B; WHO/Food Add./66.25, 1966, p. 104.
5. WHO/IARC Monographs on the evaluation of carcinogenic risk of chemicals to man. International Agency for Research on Cancer, Lyon, France, Vol. 16, 1978, p. 146.
6. Ref. 1, p. 15.
7. Ref. 5, p. 150.
8. Ref. 5, p. 145.
9. Ref. 2, p. 147.
10. Ref. 3, p. 9.
11. Ref. 2, p. 126.
12. WHO/FAO. Specifications for identity and purity of food additives (Food Colours). Fourth report. (Subsequently revised and published as Specifications for Identity and Purity of Food Additives, Vol. II. Food Colours) Rome, Food and Agriculture Organization of the United Nations, 1963, p. 35.
13. Ref. 2, p. 163.
14. Ref. 1, p. 13.
15. WHO/FAO. Evaluation of certain food additives. 21st Report of the Joint FAO/WHO Expert Committee on Food Additives. Wld. Hlth. Org. Techn. Rep. Ser., No. 617, 1978, p. 15.
16. Ref. 15, pp. 15, 37.
17. WHO/FAO. Toxicological evaluation of some food colours, enzymes, flavour enhancers, thickening agents, and certain other food additives. FAO Nutrition Meeting Report Series, No. 55; WHO Food Additives Series, No. 6, 1975, p. 38.
18. WHO/FAO. Evaluation of certain food additives. 18th report of the Joint FAO/WHO Expert Committee on Food Additives. FAO Nutrition Meetings Report Series, No. 54; Wld. Hlth. Org. Techn. Rep. Ser., No. 557, 1974, p. 15.
19. Ref. 15, p. 15.
20. Ref. 17, p. 41.
21. Ref. 15, pp. 15, 40.
22. Ref. 15, p. 15.
23. WHO/FAO. Summary of toxicological data of certain food additives. WHO Food Additives Series No. 12, 1978.
24. WHO/IARC. Monographs on the evaluation of carcinogenic risk of chemicals to man: some aromatic azo compounds. International Agency for Research on Cancer, Lyon, France, Vol. 8, 1975, pp. 42-43.
25. Ref. 4, p. 25.
26. WHO/FAO. Evaluation of mercury, lead, cadmium, and the food additives amaranth, diethylpyrocarbonate and octyl gallate. FAO Nutrition Meetings Report Series, No. 51A; WHO Food Additives Series, No. 4, pp. 64-65, 1972. 16th report of the Joint FAO/WHO Expert Committee

on Food Additives. FAO Nutrition Meetings Report Series, No. 51, Wld. Hlth. Org. Techn. Rep. Ser. No. 505, 1972, pp. 24, 32.

27. WHO/FAO. Toxicological evaluation of some food colours, thickening agents, and certain other substances, FAO Nutrition Meetings Report Series, No. 55A; WHO Food Additives Series, No. 8, 1975, pp. 24-25.

28. Ref. 24, p. 41.

29. Ref. 27, p. 20.

30. WHO/FAO. Evaluation of certain food additives: some food colours thickening agents, smoke condensates, and certain other substances. 19th report of the Joint FAO/WHO Expert Committee on Food Additives. FAO Nutrition Meetings Report Series, No. 55; Wld. Hlth. Org. Techn. Rep. Ser., No. 576, p. 14, 1975.

31. Ref. 27, p. 20.

32. Ref. 30, p. 23.

33. Ref. 2, p. 51.

34. Ref. 4, p. 22.

35. Ref. 26, p. 60.

36. Ref. 27, p. 10.

37. Ref. 24, p. 41.

38. Ref. 12, p. 69.

39. WHO/FAO. Toxicological evaluation of certain food additives. 22nd report of the Joint FAO/WHO Expert Committee on Food Additives. Wld. Hlth. Org. Techn. Rep. Ser., (to be published), 1978.

40. WHO/FAO. Toxicological evaluation of certain food additives (summaries of toxicological studies). WHO Food Additives Series No. (to be issued), 1978.

41. Ref. 12, p. 49.

42. WHO/FAO. Specifications for the identity and purity of some food colours, flavour enhancers, thickening agents, and certain other food additives. FAO Nutrition Meetings Report Series, No. 54B; WHO Food Additives Series, No. 7, 1976, p. 5.

43. WHO/FAO. Specifications for the identity and purity of food additives and their toxicological evaluation: some food colours, emulsifiers, stabilizers, anti-caking agents, and certain other substances. 13th report of the Joint FAO/WHO Expert Committee on Food Additives. FAO Nutrition Meetings Report Series, No. 46; Wld. Hlth Org. Techn. Rep. Ser., No. 445, 1970, pp. 10-11, 32.

44. WHO/FAO. Toxicological evaluation of some food colours, emulsifiers, stabilizers, anti-caking agents, and certain other substances. FAO Nutrition Meetings Report Series, No. 46A; WHO/Food Add./70.36, 1970, p. 13.

45. Ref. 18, pp. 15, and 33.

46. Ref. 17, p. 46.

47. Ref. 18, p. 36.

48. Ref. 2, p. 165.

49. Ref. 44, p. 11.

50. Ref. 17, p. 43.

51. Ref. 12, p. 48.

52. WHO/FAO. Specifications for the identity and purity of some food colours, emulsifiers, stabilizers, anti-caking agents, and certain other food additives. FAO Nutrition Meetings Report Series, No. 46B; WHO/Food Add./70.37, 1970. p. 2.

53. Ref. 42, p. 4.

54. Ref. 12, p. 38.

55. Ref. 12, p. 39.

56. Ref. 15, p. 15.

57. WHO/IARC. Monographs on the evaluation of carcinogenic risk of chemicals to man. International Agency for Research on Cancer, Lyon, France, Vol. 1, 1972, p. 70.
58. Ref. 4, p. 15.
59. Ref. 1, p. 21.
60. Ref. 3.
61. Ref. 57, p. 72.
62. Ref. 57, p. 69.
63. Ref. 2, p. 100.
64. Ref. 24, pp. 84-85.
65. Ref. 17, pp. 49-50.
66. CEC. Reports of the Scientific Committee for Food. First Series. Commission of the European Communities, December 31, 1975, p. 24.
67. Ref. 24, p. 87.
68. Ref. 18, pp. 15, 36.
69. Ref. 17, p. 50.
70. Ref. 2, p. 47.
71. Ref. 17, p. 47.
72. Ref. 24, p. 83.
73. Ref. 12, p. 71.
74. Ref. 4, p. 105.
75. Ref. 42, p. 11.
76. Ref. 66, pp. 18, 28.
77. Ref. 66, pp. 18, 27.
78. Ref. 66, pp. 17, 24.
79. Ref. 66, pp. 18, 26.
80. Ref. 12, p. 41.
81. Ref. 42, p. 14.
82. Ref. 18, pp. 15, 33.
83. Ref. 17, p. 52.
84. Ref. 18, p. 36.
85. Ref. 17, p. 51.
86. Ref. 12, p. 41.
87. Ref. 2, p. 174.
88. Ref. 5, p. 155.
89. Ref. 5, p. 159.
90. Ref. 15, pp. 15, 16.
91. Ref. 5, p. 153.
92. Ref. 12, p. 115.
93. Ref. 4, p. 107.
94. Ref. 2, p. 122.
95. Ref. 4, p. 109.
96. Ref. 1, pp. 14, 21.
97. Ref. 4, p. 109.
98. WHO/FAO. Specifications for the identity and purity of food additives and their toxicological evaluation; some emulsifiers and stabilizers and certain other substances. 10th report of the Joint FAO/WHO Expert Committee on Food Additives. FAO Nutrition Meetings Report Series, No. 43; Wld. Hlth. Org. Techn. Rep. Ser., No. 373, 1967, pp. 22 and 27.
99. Ref. 15, p. 16.
100. Ref. 4, p. 109.
101. Ref. 4, p. 110.
102. Ref. 5, p. 165.
103. Ref. 5, p. 163.
104. Ref. 5, pp. 165-166.
105. Ref. 4, p. 110.

106. Ref. 5, p. 168.
107. Ref. 1, p. 114.
108. Ref. 43, pp. 12, 32.
109. Ref. 44, p. 29.
110. Ref. 17, p. 55.
111. Ref. 18, pp. 15, 33.
112. Ref. 2, p. 90.
113. Ref. 44, p. 28.
114. Ref. 17, p. 53.
115. Ref. 12, p. 117.
116. Ref. 4, p. 112.
117. Ref. 42, p. 28.
118. Ref. 5, p. 171.
119. Ref. 5, p. 175.
120. Ref. 5, p. 176.
121. Ref. 4, p. 30.
122. Ref. 43, p. 12.
123. Ref. 44, p. 26.
124. Ref. 43, p. 32.
125. Ref. 5, p. 182.
126. Ref. 2, p. 112.
127. Ref. 4, p. 28.
128. Ref. 44, p. 24.
129. Ref. 12, p. 107.
130. Ref. 4, p. 27.
131. Ref. 4, p. 114.
132. Ref. 15, p. 16.
133. Ref. 66, pp. 19, 25.
134. Ref. 2, p. 73.
135. Ref. 24, p. 126.
136. Ref. 1, p. 21.
137. Ref. 4, p. 13.
138. Ref. 2, p. 8.
139. Ref. 24, pp. 137-138.
140. Ref. 24, p. 125.
141. Ref. 17, p. 57.
142. Ref. 42, p. 31.
143. Ref. 4, p. 33.
144. Ref. 98, pp. 22, 27.
145. WHO/FAO. Toxicological evaluation of certain food additives with a
     review of general principles and of specifications. 17th report of
     the Joint FAO/WHO Expert Committee on Food Additives, FAO Nutrition
     Meetings Report Series, No. 53; Wld. Hlth. Org. Techn. Rep. Ser.,
     No. 539, 1974, p. 11.
146. Ref. 18, pp. 15, 33.
147. Ref. 17, p. 58.
148. Ref. 66, pp. 17, 23.
149. Ref. 4, p. 32.
150. Ref. 4, p. 31.
151. Ref. 15, p. 16.
152. Ref. 43, p. 11.
153. WHO/FAO. Evaluation of food additives. 15th report of the Joint
     FAO/WHO Expert Committee on Food Additives. FAO Nutrition Meetings
     Report Series, No. 50; Wld. Hlth. Org. Techn. Rep. Ser., No. 488,
     1972, p. 16.
154. Ref. 17, p. 59.

155. WHO/FAO. Evaluation of certain food additives and the contaminants
     mercury, lead, and cadmium. 16th report of the Joint FAO/WHO Ex-
     pert Committee on Food Additives. FAO Nutrition Meetings Report
     Series, No. 51; Wld. Hlth. Org. Techn. Rep. Ser., No. 505, 1972,
     p. 25.
156. Ref. 43, pp. 11-12.
157. Ref. 42, p. 12.
158. Ref. 153, pp. 15-16, 41.
159. WHO/FAO. Toxicological evaluation of some enzymes, modified starches,
     and certain other substances. FAO Nutrition Meetings Report Series,
     No. 50A; WHO Food Additives Series, No. 1., 1972, p. 65.
160. Ref. 18, pp. 16, 33.
161. Ref. 17, p. 63.
162. Ref. 15, pp. 16, 17.
163. Ref. 66, pp. 17, 23, 25.
164. Ref. 149, p. 61.
165. Ref. 23, (to be issued).
166. WHO/FAO. Specifications for the identity and purity of some en-
     zymes and certain other substances. FAO Nutrition Meetings Report
     Series, No. 50B; WHO Food Additives Series, No. 2, 1972, pp. 30,
     33.
167. Ref. 42, p. 35.
168. FAO/WHO. Specifications for identity and purity of some food addi-
     tives, including antioxidants, food colours, thickeners, and others.
     FAO Nutrition Meetings Report Series, No. 57, 1977, p. 8.
169. Ref. 2, p. 17.
170. Ref. 15, pp. 17, 18.
171. Ref. 66, p. 18.
172. Ref. 42, pp. 16-17.
173. Ref. 17, p. 65.
174. Ref. 4, p. 37.
175. Ref. 98, pp. 22, 27.
176. Ref. 145, p. 11.
177. Ref. 98, p. 22.
178. Ref. 18, pp. 16, 33.
179. Ref. 17, p. 67.
180. Ref. 4, p. 36.
181. Ref. 4, p. 34.
182. Ref. 42, p. 16.
183. Ref. 42, p. 18.
184. Ref. 12, p. 56.
185. Ref. 2, p. 171.
186. Ref. 12, p. 46.
187. Ref. 42, p. 24.
188. Ref. 4, p. 41.
189. Ref. 98, pp. 22, 27.
190. Ref. 17, p. 71.
191. Ref. 17, p. 70.
192. Ref. 4, p. 40.
193. Ref. 17, p. 68.
194. Ref. 12, p. 45.
195. Ref. 4, p. 38.
196. Ref. 42, p. 24.
197. Ref. 42, p. 25.
198. Ref. 42, pp. 20-21.
199. Ref. 4, p. 45.
200. Ref. 17, p. 72.

201. Ref. 17, p. 73.
202. Ref. 4, p. 44.
203. Ref. 4, p. 43.
204. Ref. 42, p. 22.
205. Ref. 2, p. 174.
206. Ref. 15, p. 18.
207. Ref. 52, p. 9.
208. Ref. 43, p. 11.
209. Ref. 44, p. 14.
210. Ref. 12, p. 63.
211. Ref. 52, p. 7.
212. Ref. 2, p. 170.
213. Ref. 52, p. 9.
214. Ref. 42, p. 44.
215. Ref. 44, p. 16-17.
216. Ref. 44, p. 17.
217. Ref. 18, p. 16.
218. Ref. 17, p. 77.
219. Ref. 66, pp. 17, 23.
220. Ref. 44, p. 15.
221. Ref. 12, p. 65.
222. Ref. 52, p. 10.
223. Ref. 42, p. 44.
224. Ref. 42, p. 47.
225. Ref. 44, pp. 16-17.
226. Ref. 17, p. 76.
227. Ref. 44, p. 17.
228. Ref. 17, p. 77.
229. Ref. 18, p. 17.
230. Ref. 15, pp. 28-29, 37.
231. Ref. 44, p. 15.
232. Ref. 17, p. 74.
233. Ref. 12, p. 65.
234. Ref. 52, p. 12.
235. Ref. 42, p. 47.
236. Ref. 15, p. 18.
237. Ref. 2, p. 92.
238. Ref. 4, p. 115.
239. Ref. 15, p. 18.
240. Ref. 66, pp. 18, 25.
241. Ref. 4, p. 115.
242. Ref. 2, p. 93.
243. Ref. 4, p. 116.
244. Ref. 4, p. 154.
245. Ref. 24, p. 92.
246. Ref. 4, p. 16.
247. Ref. 1, p. 22.
248. Ref. 24, p. 94.
249. Ref. 24, p. 91.
250. Ref. 2, p. 9.
251. Ref. 4, p. 117.
252. Ref. 14, p. 18.
253. Ref. 66, pp. 18-19, 28.
254. Ref. 4, p. 118.
255. Ref. 12, p. 90.
256. Ref. 4, pp. 118, 154.
257. Ref. 2, p. 41.

258. Ref. 2, p. 61.
259. Kolk, J.H.H. About Vitamin A efficiency and pigmenting effect of three citranaxanthin preparations at chicks and quails with different crystal size. Dissertation, University Munich, 1974.
260. Kawase, S., Komatsu, Y., Suzuki, Y., Nishida, S., and Kobayshi, A. Subacute toxicity of citranaxanthin, J. Med. Soc., Toho, Japan, 19, 1972, pp. 499-504.
261. Ref. 168, p. 153.
262. Ref. 168, p. 10.
263. Ref. 168, p. 14.
264. Ref. 168, p. 17.
265. Ref. 168, pp. 149, 153.
266. Ref. 168, p. 22.
267. Ref. 168, pp. 30, 42, 50.
268. Ref. 168, pp. 55, 58.
269. Ref. 168, p. 60.
270. Ref. 168, p. 61.
271. Ref. 168, p. 63.
272. Ref. 168, p. 153.
273. Ref. 168, p. 65.
274. Ref. 24, p. 102.
275. Ref. 44, p. 32.
276. Ref. 43, pp. 12-13.
277. Ref. 4, p. 47.
278. Ref. 44, p. 30.
279. Ref. 24, p. 101.
280. Ref. 4, p. 46.
281. Ref. 12, p. 43.
282. Ref. 168, p. 52.
283. Ref. 15, pp. 18, 19.
284. Ref. 18, pp. 17, 33.
285. Ref. 66, pp. 18, 28.
286. Ref. 17, p. 78.
287. Ref. 12, p. 43.
288. Ref. 168, p. 52.
289. Ref. 168, p. 54.
290. Ref. 2, p. 162.
291. Ref. 4, p. 17.
292. Ref. 3, p. 89.
293. Ref. 2, p. 85.
294. WHO/IARC. Monographs on the evaluation of carcinogenic risk of chemicals to man: some fumigants, the herbicides 2,4-d, and 2,4,5-T chlorinated dibenzodioxins and miscellaneous industrial chemicals. International Agency for Research on Cancer, Lyon, France, Vol. 15, 1977, pp. 186-187.
295. Ref. 4, p. 119.
296. Ref. 2, p. 140.
297. Ref. 3, p. 96.
298. Ref. 294, p. 190.
299. Ref. 1, p. 22.
300. Ref. 4, p. 17.
301. Ref. 43, pp. 12, 32.
302. Ref. 44, p. 36.
303. Ref. 18, pp. 17, 34.
304. Ref. 17, p. 86.
305. Ref. 4, p. 52.
306. Ref. 44, p. 33.

307. Ref. 17, p. 80.
308. Ref. 12, p. 83.
309. Ref. 4, p. 50.
310. Ref. 52, p. 14.
311. Ref. 42, p. 50.
312. Ref. 4, p. 51.
313. Ref. 52, p. 16.
314. Ref. 42, p. 51.
315. Ref. 2, p. 143.
316. Ref. 4, p. 15.
317. Ref. 1, p. 22.
318. Ref. 5, pp. 189, 190.
319. Ref. 44, p. 39.
320. Ref. 43, pp. 12, 32.
321. Ref. 5, p. 194.
322. Ref. 4, p. 57.
323. Ref. 44, p. 38.
324. Ref. 5, p. 187.
325. Ref. 12, p. 99.
326. Ref. 4, p. 5.
327. Ref. 5, pp. 190-191.
328. Ref. 2, p. 131.
329. Ref. 1, p. 22.
330. Ref. 4, pp. 17, 120.
331. Ref. 2, p. 49.
332. Ref. 3, p. 101.
333. Ref. 15, p. 19.
334. Ref. 66, pp. 18, 28.
335. Ref. 12, p. 73.
336. Ref. 4, p. 120.
337. Ref. 168, p. 71.
338. Ref. 168, p. 153.
339. Ref. 2, p. 49.
340. Ref. 4, pp. 17, 122.
341. Ref. 2, pp. 5-6.
342. Ref. 3, p. 110.
343. Ref. 15, p. 19.
344. Ref. 12, p. 92.
345. Ref. 4, p. 122.
346. Ref. 4, p. 123.
347. Ref. 2, p. 5.
348. Ref. 27, p. 3.
349. Ref. 18, pp. 17, 34, 36.
350. Ref. 18, pp. 24, 35.
351. Ref. 17, p. 182.
352. Ref. 30, pp. 14, 21.
353. Ref. 27, p. 27.
354. Ref. 27, p. 26.
355. Ref. 42, p. 169.
356. Ref. 42, p. 171.
357. Ref. 4, p. 17.
358. Ref. 2, p. 139.
359. Ref. 3, p. 104.
360. Ref. 43, p. 12.
361. Ref. 42, p. 53.
362. Ref. 1, p. 24.
363. Ref. 4, pp. 20, 99.

364. Ref. 43, pp. 12, 32.
365. Ref. 44, p. 59.
366. Ref. 18, pp. 17, 34.
367. Ref. 17, p. 92.
368. Ref. 66, pp. 18, 25.
369. Ref. 4, p. 99.
370. Ref. 43, p. 57.
371. Ref. 17, p. 89.
372. Ref. 12, p. 105.
373. Ref. 4, pp. 99-100.
374. Ref. 42, p. 55.
375. Ref. 168, p. 73.
376. Ref. 4, p. 154.
377. Ref. 168, pp. 149, 153.
378. Ref. 2, p. 130.
379. Ref. 1, p. 22.
380. Ref. 4, p. 17.
381. Ref. 15, p. 19.
382. Ref. 66, pp. 18, 27.
383. Ref. 2, p. 106.
384. Ref. 5, p. 205.
385. Ref. 5, p. 199.
386. Ref. 12, p. 101.
387. Ref. 98, p. 22.
388. Ref. 43, pp. 12, 32.
389. Ref. 44, p. 42.
390. Ref. 17, p. 194.
391. Ref. 66, pp. 18, 29.
392. Ref. 4, p. 60.
393. Ref. 44, p. 41.
394. Ref. 17, p. 93.
395. Ref. 12, p. 113.
396. Ref. 4, pp. 60-61.
397. Ref. 4, p. 154.
398. Ref. 2, p. 155.
399. Ref. 43, pp. 12, 32.
400. Ref. 44, p. 45.
401. Ref. 18, pp. 17, 34.
402. Ref. 17, p. 99.
403. Ref. 17, p. 98.
404. Ref. 66, pp. 17, 23.
405. Ref. 4, p. 63.
406. Ref. 44, p. 43.
407. Ref. 17, p. 95.
408. Ref. 12, p. 63.
409. Ref. 42, p. 58.
410. Ref. 4, p. 154.
411. Ref. 42, p. 60.
412. Ref. 2, p. 157.
413. Ref. 42, pp. 61-62.
414. Ref. 18, pp. 17, 34, 36.
415. Ref. 17, p. 101.
416. Ref. 66, pp. 17, 24.
417. Ref. 17, p. 100.
418. Ref. 57, p. 29.
419. Ref. 12, p. 19.
420. Ref. 42, p. 61.

421. Ref. 42, p. 62.
422. Ref. 1, p. 22.
423. Ref. 4, pp. 17, 125.
424. Ref. 1, p. 24.
425. Ref. 5, pp. 210-211.
426. Ref. 5, p. 216.
427. Ref. 5, p. 209.
428. Ref. 12, p. 103.
429. Ref. 4, p. 125.
430. Ref. 2, p. 108.
431. Ref. 15, p. 19.
432. Ref. 66, pp. 18, 28.
433. Ref. 168, p. 84.
434. Ref. 168, p. 153.
435. Ref. 18, pp. 17-18.
436. Ref. 15, p. 20.
437. Ref. 66, pp. 18, 26-27.
438. Ref. 1, p. 23.
439. Ref. 4, p. 18.
440. WHO/IARC. Monographs on the evaluation of carcinogenic risk of
     chemicals to man: some aromatic amines, hydrazine, and related
     substances, N-nitroso compounds and miscellaneous alkylating agents.
     International Agency for Research on Cancer, Lyon France, Vol. 4,
     1974, pp. 60-61.
441. Ref. 440, p. 63.
442. Ref. 440, p. 57.
443. Ref. 2, p. 116.
444. Ref. 3, p. 134.
445. Ref. 2, p. 102.
446. Ref. 3, p. 138.
447. Ref. 2, p. 40.
448. Ref. 4, pp. 18, 127.
449. Ref. 4, p. 127.
450. Ref. 2, p. 117.
451. Ref. 3, p. 142.
452. Ref. 2, p. 77.
453. Ref. 2, p. 2.
454. Ref. 4, p. 128.
455. Ref. 3, p. 145.
456. Ref. 2, p. 152.
457. Ref. 24, pp. 166-167.
458. Ref. 2, p. 69.
459. Ref. 24, p. 169.
460. Ref. 24, p. 165.
461. Ref. 24, p. 233.
462. Ref. 24, pp. 234-235.
463. Ref. 4, pp. 13, 18.
464. Ref. 2, p. 27.
465. Ref. 24, p. 237.
466. Ref. 24, p. 233.
467. Ref. 2, p. 10.
468. Ref. 24, p. 283.
469. Ref. 2, p. 11.
470. Ref. 24, p. 279.
471. Ref. 24, pp. 288-289.
472. Ref. 2, p. 24.
473. Ref. 24, p. 291.

474. Ref. 24, p. 287.
475. WHO/FAO. Specifications for the identity and purity of some ex-
     traction solvents and certain other substances. FAO Nutrition
     Meetings Report Series, No. 48B; WHO/Food Add./70.40, 1971, p. 25.
476. WHO/FAO, Toxicological evaluation of some extraction solvents and
     certain other substances. FAO Nutrition Meetings Report Series, No.
     48A; WHO/Food Add./70.39, 1971, p. 60.
477. WHO/FAO. Evaluation of food additives. 14th report of the Joint
     FAO/WHO Expert Committee on Food Additives. FAO Nutrition Meetings
     Report Series, No. 48; Wld. Hlth. Org. Techn. Rep. Ser., No. 462,
     1971, pp. 23, 24.
478. Ref. 18, p. 10.
479. Ref. 24, p. 174.
480. Ref. 4, p. 69.
481. Ref. 44, p. 47.
482. Ref. 43, p. 12.
483. Ref. 15, p. 20.
484. Ref. 24, p. 177.
485. Ref. 4, p. 68.
486. Ref. 44, p. 46.
487. Ref. 24, p. 173.
488. Ref. 4, pp. 67-68.
489. Ref. 2, p. 43.
490. Ref. 2, p. 44.
491. Ref. 24, pp. 182-183.
492. Ref. 4, pp. 18, 130.
493. Ref. 24, p. 185.
494. Ref. 66, pp. 18, 29.
495. Ref. 24, p. 181.
496. Ref. 4, p. 130.
497. Ref. 2, p. 18.
498. Ref. 4, pp. 18, 133.
499. Ref. 2, p. 63.
500. Ref. 18, p. 18.
501. Ref. 15, p. 20.
502. Ref. 12, p. 86.
503. Ref. 4, p. 133.
504. Ref. 17, p. 104.
505. Ref. 18, pp. 18, 34.
506. Ref. 15, p. 20.
507. Ref. 17, p. 102.
508. Ref. 2, p. 16.
509. Ref. 12, p. 67.
510. Ref. 18, pp. 18, 34.
511. Ref. 2, p. 166.
512. Ref. 4, pp. 19, 71.
513. Ref. 44, p. 50.
514. Ref. 43, pp. 12, 32.
515. Ref. 17, p. 108.
516. Ref. 18, pp. 18, 34.
517. Ref. 66, pp. 18, 25.
518. Ref. 4, p. 71.
519. Ref. 44, p. 49.
520. Ref. 17, p. 106.
521. Ref. 12, p. 109.
522. Ref. 4, p. 71.
523. Ref. 42, p. 67.

524. Ref. 108, p. 92.
525. Ref. 42, p. 69.
526. Ref. 108, pp. 149, 1953.
527. Ref. 2, p. 115.
528. Ref. 2, p. 160.
529. Ref. 15, p. 20.
530. Ref. 24, pp. 190-191.
531. Ref. 4, pp. 19, 135.
532. Ref. 2, p. 32.
533. Ref. 24, p. 195.
534. Ref. 24, p. 189.
535. Ref. 4, p. 135.
536. Ref. 24, pp. 200-201.
537. Ref. 4, pp. 13, 19.
538. Ref. 2, p. 34.
539. Ref. 24, p. 204.
540. Ref. 24, p. 199.
541. Ref. 4, pp. 19, 74.
542. Ref. 44, p. 52.
543. Ref. 43, pp. 12, 32.
544. Ref. 17, p. 112.
545. Ref. 18, pp. 18, 34.
546. Ref. 18, p. 36.
547. Ref. 4, p. 74.
548. Ref. 44, p. 51.
549. Ref. 17, p. 109.
550. Ref. 12, p. 75.
551. Ref. 4, p. 74.
552. Ref. 42, p. 70.
553. Ref. 168, p. 95.
554. Ref. 42, p. 71.
555. Ref. 168, pp. 149, 153.
556. Ref. 2, p. 53.
557. Ref. 4, pp. 19, 137.
558. Ref. 17, p. 114.
559. Ref. 15, pp. 20, 21.
560. Ref. 17, p. 113.
561. Ref. 12, p. 77.
562. Ref. 4, p. 138.
563. Ref. 2, p. 55.
564. Ref. 24, pp. 208-209.
565. Ref. 2, p. 66.
566. Ref. 16.
567. Ref. 24, pp. 212-213.
568. Ref. 24, p. 207.
569. Ref. 12, p. 79.
570. Ref. 2, p. 175.
571. Ref. 4, pp. 19, 77.
572. Ref. 43, p. 32.
573. Ref. 44, p. 18.
574. Ref. 15, p. 21.
575. Ref. 4, p. 78.
576. Ref. 42, p. 73.
577. Ref. 27, p. 30.
578. Ref. 4, p. 81.
579. Ref. 44, p. 53.
580. Ref. 17, p. 116.

581. Ref. 27, p. 28.
582. Ref. 12, p. 97.
583. Ref. 4, p. 80.
584. Ref. 168, p. 98.
585. Ref. 168, p. 149.
586. Ref. 2, p. 149.
587. Ref. 4, pp. 19, 140.
588. Ref. 3, p. 203.
589. Ref. 4, p. 140.
590. Ref. 2, p. 19.
591. Ref. 1, p. 24.
592. Ref. 4, pp. 19, 143.
593. Ref. 15, p. 21.
594. Ref. 4, p. 143.
595. Ref. 108, p. 100.
596. Ref. 108, pp. 149, 153.
597. Ref. 2, p. 21.
598. Ref. 4, p. 19.
599. Ref. 3, p. 209.
600. Ref. 4, p. 19, 146.
601. Ref. 3, p. 211.
602. Ref. 2, p. 135.
603. Ref. 5, pp. 224-225.
604. Ref. 5, p. 228.
605. Ref. 5, p. 221.
606. Ref. 4, p. 146.
607. Ref. 3, p. 218.
608. Ref. 2, p. 137.
609. Ref. 5, p. 235.
610. Ref. 5, p. 237.
611. Ref. 5, p. 233.
612. Ref. 12, p. 57.
613. Ref. 98, p. 22.
614. Ref. 43, pp. 11, 32.
615. Ref. 44, p. 21.
616. Ref. 44, p. 20.
617. Ref. 2, p. 173.
618. Ref. 15, pp. 20, 21.
619. Ref. 168, p. 102.
620. Ref. 12, p. 51.
621. Ref. 2, p. 167.
622. Ref. 4, pp. 19, 148.
623. Ref. 3, p. 226.
624. Ref. 2, p. 68.
625. Ref. 15, p. 22.
626. Ref. 12, p. 81.
627. Ref. 4, p. 148.
628. Ref. 15, p. 22.
629. Ref. 2, p. 15.
630. Ref. 4, p. 13, 20.
631. Ref. 24, p. 226.
632. Ref. 24, p. 229.
633. Ref. 24, p. 225.
634. Ref. 4, p. 20.
635. Ref. 2, p. 78.
636. Ref. 24, pp. 242-243.
637. Ref. 24, p. 245.

638. Ref. 24, p. 241.
639. Ref. 3, p. 238.
640. Ref. 2, p. 80.
641. Ref. 24, pp. 218-219.
642. Ref. 24, p. 222.
643. Ref. 24, p. 217.
644. Ref. 3, p. 242.
645. Ref. 2, p. 13.
646. Ref. 4, p. 150.
647. Ref. 4, pp. 20, 151.
648. Ref. 3, p. 245.
649. Ref. 2, p. 39.
650. Ref. 4, p. 150.
651. Ref. 24, pp. 258-259.
652. Ref. 4, p. 86.
653. Ref. 1, p. 14.
654. Ref. 24, p. 263.
655. Ref. 4, p. 83.
656. Ref. 24, p. 257.
657. Ref. 12, p. 88.
658. Ref. 2, p. 58.
659. Ref. 1, pp. 14, 24.
660. Ref. 4, pp. 12, 20, 92.
661. Ref. 4, p. 92.
662. Ref. 4, p. 88.
663. Ref. 12, p. 95.
664. Ref. 2, p. 99.
665. Ref. 3, p. 259.
666. Ref. 2, p. 91.
667. Ref. 4, p. 20, 93.
668. Ref. 43, pp. 13, 32.
669. Ref. 44, p. 56.
670. Ref. 4, p. 96.
671. Ref. 44, p. 55.
672. Ref. 12, p. 24.
673. Ref. 4, p. 93.
674. Ref. 4, p. 94.
675. Ref. 42, p. 75.
676. Ref. 475, p. 9.
677. Ref. 43, pp. 11, 32.
678. Ref. 44, p. 23.
679. Ref. 43, p. 11.
680. Ref. 18, pp. 19, 34.
681. Ref. 17, p. 121.
682. Ref. 18, p. 19.
683. Ref. 18, pp. 36-37.
684. Ref. 12, p. 60.
685. Ref. 475, pp. 9, 32.
686. Ref. 475. p. 33.
687. Ref. 42, p. 76.
688. Ref. 475, p. 10.
689. Ref. 2, p. 161.
690. Ref. 12, p. 30.
691. Ref. 15, p. 22.
692. Ref. 3, p. 271.
693. Ref. 3, p. 273.
694. Ref. 4, p. 152.

695. Ref. 2, p. 124.
696. Ref. 3, p. 275.
697. Ref. 2, p. 127.
698. Ref. 12, p. 56.
699. Ref. 15, pp. 22, 23.
700. Ref. 12, p. 55.
701. Ref. 43, p. 12.
702. Ref. 18, pp. 18, 24.
703. Ref. 17, p. 123.
704. Ref. 15, p. 22.
705. Ref. 17, p. 122.
706. Ref. 168, p. 147.
707. Ref. 168, pp. 149, 153.
708. Ref. 2, p. 97.
709. Ref. 4, pp. 20, 153.
710. Ref. 3, p. 278.
711. Ref. 2, p. 59.
712. FAO. Specifications, identity and purity of certain food additives (to be published), 1978.
713. CEC. Report of the Scientific Committee for Food. Fourth Series. Commission of the European Communities, December 1977, p. 28.
714. Ref. 722, p. 29.
715. Ref. 722, p. 30.

TABLE I

Listing of Food Colorants and Their Toxicological Assessment

Compound	Maximum acceptable daily intake for man (mg/kg bw) and other toxicological decisions	Remarks
Aluminium	-	The use is very limited; not considered to present a hazard (1)
Amaranth	0.75	Temporary evaluation: The compound is scheduled for reevaluation in 1982 (2)
Annatto	1.25	Expressed as bixin; temporary evaluation: This substance is scheduled for reevaluation in 1978 (3)
Auramine	"Not to be used"	Colorant found to be harmful (4)
Azorubine	1.25	Temporary evaluation: The compound is scheduled for reevaluation in 1982 (2)
Beet red	"ADI not specified"	Temporary evaluation: This colorant is scheduled for reevaluation in 1982 (2)
Benzyl violet 4B	"Not to be used"	The safety of this colorant has not been satisfactorily established (5)
Brilliant black PN	2.5	Temporary evaluation: The compound is scheduled for reevaluation in 1981 (2)

TABLE I Cont.

Brilliant Blue FCF	12.5	This colorant has a fixed ADI (6)
Butter yellow	"Not to be used"	Colorant found to be harmful (4)
Canthaxanthine	25	This colorant has a fixed ADI (7)
Caramel (ammonia-sulfite)	100	Temporary evaluation: These substances are scheduled to be reevaluated in 1980 (8)
Caramel (not ammoniated)	"ADI not specified"	These products have a fixed ADI (9)
β-apo-8' carotenal	5	Group ADI; as the sum of β-carotene, β-apo-8'-carotenal, and β-apo-8' carotenic acid, ethyl, and methyl esters (10)
β-carotene (synthetic)	5	Group ADI (10)
β-apo-8'-carotenoic acid, ethyl, and methyl esters	5	Group ADI (10)
Chlorophyll copper complex	15	This complex has a fixed ADI (11)
Chlorophyllin copper complex, sodium, and potassium salts	15	The previous temporary ADI was converted to an ADI (12)
Chlorophylls	"ADI not specified"	These products have a fixed ADI (11)

Compound	ADI	Evaluation
Chocolate brown HT	0.25	Temporary evaluation: The compound is scheduled for reevaluation in 1979 (13)
Chrysoidine	"Not to be used"	Colorant found to be harmful (14)
Citrus red No. 2	"Not to be used"	Information was not sufficient to establish its safety in use (15)
Curcumin	0.1	Temporary evaluation: The compound is scheduled for reevaluation in 1980 (2)
Erythrosine	2.5	This colorant has a fixed ADI. A limit of 0.1% fluoresceine was established (16)
Fast green FCF	12.5	This compound has a fixed ADI (17)
Ferrous gluconate (coloring agent)	"ADI not specified"	Evaluation relates to its use as coloring adjunct and not as a nutritional supplement with the proviso that the contribution from ferrous gluconate to the total dietary gluconic acid intake from all sources should be included in the ADI for gluconic acid (50 mg/kg bw) (18)
Fluoresceine	"Not to be used"	Information is not sufficient for evaluation but indicates possibility of harmful effects (14)

TABLE I Cont.

Food green S	—	Previously referred to as wool green BS[19] and green S[20]; the temporary ADI was revoked (20)
Gold	—	The use is very limited; Not considered to present a hazard (21)
Guinea green B	"Not to be used"	Colorant harmful (14)
Indanthrene blue RS	—	Previous temporary ADI was revoked (22)
Indigotine	5	This compound has a fixed ADI (22)
Iron oxides/hydrated iron oxides	"Not to be used"	Temporary evaluation: These compounds are scheduled for reevaluation in 1979 (2)
Light green SF	"Not to be used"	Information is not sufficient for evaluation, but indicates possibility of harmful effects (14)
Magenta	"Not to be used"	Colorant found to be harmful (23)
Malachite green	"Not to be used"	Information is not sufficient for evaluation but indicates possibility of harmful effects (23)
Nigrosine	"Not to be used"	Information is not sufficient for evaluation but indicates possibility of harmful effects (23)
Oil orange SS	"Not to be used"	Colorant found to be harmful (23)

TABLE I Cont.

Oil orange XO	"Not to be used"	Colorant found to be harmful (23)
Oil yellow AB	"Not to be used"	Colorant found to be harmful (23)
Oil yellow OB	"Not to be used"	Colorant found to be harmful (23)
Patent blue V	-	Previous temporary ADI was revoked (24)
Ponceau 2R (MX)	"Not to be used"	Information is not sufficient for evaluation, but indicates possibility of harmful effects (23)
Ponceau 3R	"Not to be used"	Colorant found to be harmful (23)
Ponceau 4R	0.125	Temporary evaluation: The compound is scheduled for reevaluation in 1981 (1)
Ponceau SX	"Not to be used"	Colorant found to be harmful (23)
Quinoline yellow	0.5	Temporary evaluation: The compound is scheduled for reevaluation in 1982 (1)
Red 2G	0.006	Temporary evaluation: The compound is scheduled for reevaluation in 1979 (25)
Rhodamine B	"Not to be used"	Information is not sufficient for evaluation but indicates possibility of harmful effects (26)

TABLE I Cont.

Riboflavin	0.5	This compound has a fixed ADI (27)
Sudan I	"Not to be used"	Colorant found to be harmful (26)
Sudan IV (scarlet R)	"Not to be used"	Information is not sufficient for evaluation, but indicates possibility of harmful effects (26)
Sunset yellow FCF	5	This compound has a fixed ADI (28)
Tartrazine	7.5	This compound has a fixed ADI (28)
Titanium dioxide	"ADI not specified"	This compound has a fixed ADI (29)
Turmeric	2.5	Temporary evaluation: The compound is scheduled for reevaluation in 1980 (1)
Yellow 2G	0.025	Temporary evaluation: The compound is scheduled for reevaluation in 1979 (30)

This table reports a complete listing of food colorants for which acceptable daily intake figures (ADI's) have been established, and other toxicological decisions have been made. The listing is inclusive for compounds examined by the 1978 meeting of the Joint FAO/WHO Expert Committee on Food Additives.

Under "Remarks," brief explanatory notes are given. They are aimed at supplying exhaustive references to problems related to group evaluations, analytical aspects having a direct bearing on the ADI's, and the character of the evaluation. Dates indicating when the next reevaluation will take place are also given. In this regard, note that the document referenced after each specified data, indicating the scheduled re-evaluation, contains detailed information on the further work deemed necessary before an ADI can be recommended or confirmed.

The following toxicological decisions warrant brief explanations:

1. Temporary ADI: An acceptable daily intake may be allocated temporarily to a compound, pending the provision of additional data within a stated period of time. This measure implies that the toxicological data are adequate to ensure the safety of use of the food colorant during the time for which the temporary ADI applies. If the additional data requested do not become available within the stated period, the temporary ADI may be withdrawn.

2. ADI revoked: The ADI has been revoked either because the requested data were not submitted and no indication was given that data were forthcoming, or because the available data indicated a hazard. This fact has been often interpreted as evidence that the compound was withdrawn from marketing or production owing to lack of commercial use or interest.

3. ADI not specified: This decision means that, on the basis of the available data (toxicological, biochemical, and other) the total daily intake of the substance, arising from its use or uses at the levels necessary to achieve the desired effect and from its acceptable background of use in food, does not, in the opinion of the Committee, represent a hazard to health. For this reason, and for the reasons stated in individual evaluations, the establishment of an acceptable daily intake (ADI) in mg/kg bw is not deemed necessary.

4. Not to be used because harmful or possibly harmful. This decision is applicable to substances for which there is sufficient information on which to base such an action. Sometimes this decision is applicable to cases in which the available information is not sufficient to establish the safety in use of a compound or when the specifications for identity and purity are not adequate. The expression "not to be used" relates solely to the use in food of the compound in questions.

REFERENCES

1. Evaluation of certain food additives. Twenty-first report of the Joint FAO/WHO Expert Committee on Food Additives. Wld. Hlth. Org. Techn. Rep. Ser., No. 617, 1978, pp. 15 and 39.
2. Evaluation of certain food additives and contaminants. Twenty-second report of the Joint FAO/WHO Expert Committee on Food Additives. Wld. Hlth. Org. Techn. Rep. Ser., (In press), 1978.

3. Toxicological evaluation of certain food additives with a review of specifications. Eighteenth Report. FAO Nutrition Meetings Report Series, No. 54; Wld. Hlth. Org. Techn. Rep. Ser., No. 557, 1974, pp. 15, 33 and 36.

4. Specifications for the identity and purity of food additives and their toxicological evaluation. Food colours and some antimicrobials and antioxidants. Eighth Report. FAO Nutrition Meetings Report Series, No. 38; Wld. Hlth. Org. Techn. Rep. Ser., No. 309, 1965, p. 21.

5. Ref. 1, pp. 15-16 and 37, 39.

6. Specifications for the identity and purity of food additives and their toxicological evaluation: some food colors, emulsifiers, stabilizers, anti-caking agents, and certain other substances. Thirteenth Report. FAO Nutrition Meetings Report Series, No. 46; Wld. Hlth. Org. Techn. Rep. Ser., No. 445, 1970, p. 32.

7. Ref. 3, pp. 17 and 33.

8. Ref. 1, pp. 16-17 and 37, 40.

9. Evaluation of food additives. Some enzymes, modified starches and certain other su-stances: toxicological evaluations and specifications, and a review of the technological efficacy of some antioxidants. Fifteenth Report. FAO Nutrition Meetings Report Series, No. 50; Wld. Hlth. Org. Techn. Rep. Ser., No. 488, 1972, pp. 15-16 and 41.

10. Ref. 3, pp. 16 and 33-34.

11. Ref. 6, pp. 10 and 32.

12. Ref. 1, pp. 28-29 and 37, 39.

13. Ref. 1, pp. 18, 37, and 39-40.

14. Ref. 4, p. 22.

15. Ref. 6, pp. 12-13 and 32.

16. Ref. 3, pp. 17 and 34.

17. Ref. 6, pp. 12 and 32.

18. Evaluation of certain food additives. Nineteenth Report of the Joint FAO/WHO Expert Committee on Food Additives. FAO Nutrition Meetings Report Series, No. 55; Wld. Hlth. Org. Techn. Rep. Ser., No. 576, 1975, pp. 14 and 21.

19. Ref. 4, p. 24.

20. Ref. 3, pp. 17 and 34.

21. Ref. 1, pp. 19, 37 and 39.

22. Ref. 3, pp. 17 and 34.

23. Ref. 4, p. 23.

24. Ref. 3, pp. 18 and 34.

25. Ref. 1, pp. 21, 38 and 40.

26. Ref. 4, p. 24.

27. Ref. 6, p. 32.

28. Ref. 4, p. 14.

29. Ref. 6, pp. 13 and 32.

30. Ref. 1, pp. 22, 38 and 41.

TABLE II

Summary of Toxicological Data on Which Acceptable Daily Intake Figures are Based

Compound	Animal species	Kind of toxicological test	Levels tested	Levels causing no toxicological effects	Safety factor employed	Maximum acceptable daily intake (ADI) mg/kg bw	Brief indication of effects	References
I	II	III	IV	V	VI	VIII	VIII	IX
Amaranth	Rat	64 wk	0, 300, 3000, 15,000 ppm	3000 ppm in the diet (150 mg/kg bw)	200	0.75 (T)	Decrease in growth rate; increased weight of liver and kidneys	1 2
Annatto	Rat	2 yr	0, 500, 5000, ppm (total bixin content from 0.2 to 2.6%)	5000 ppm in the diet (250 mg/kg bw)	200	1.25 (T)	–	3 4 5
Azorubine	Rat	90-day	0, 0.005%, 0.10%, 0.50%, 1.0%	0.05% in the diet (250 mg/kg bw)	200	1.25 (T)	Elevated renal weight in female rats	2 6
Brilliant black PN	Rat	90-day	0, 3000, 10,000, 30,000 ppm	10,000 ppm in the diet (500 mg/kg bw)	200	2.5 (T)	Growth retardation; increased weight of testes and kidneys	2 7
	Rat	2 yr	0, 1000, 5000, 10,000 ppm	10,000 ppm in the diet (500 mg/kg bw)				8

Brilliant blue FCF	Rat	2 yr	0, 5000, 10,000, 20,000, 50,000 ppm	50,000 ppm in the diet (2500 mg/kg bw)	200	12.5	—	4 9
Canthaxanthine	Rat	93-98 wk	0, 5000, 20,000 50,000 ppm	50,000 ppm in the diet (2500 mg/kg bw)	100	25	—	3 10 11
Caramel (by ammonia sulfite process)	Rat	90 day	0, 50,000, 100,000, 200,000 ppm	200,000 ppm in the diet (10,000 mg/kg bw)	100	100 (T) Based on a product having a color intensity of 20,000 EBC units containing not more than 200 ppm of 4-methyl-imidazole	—	12 13
β-apo-8'-carotenal	Rat	110 wk	0, 1000 ppm	1000 ppm in the diet (50 mg/kg bw)	200	5 (as sum of β-carotene, β-apo-8'-carotenal, and β-apo-8'-caroten-oic acid, ethyl and methyl ester)	—	3
β-carotene (synthetic)	Rat	110 wk	0, 1000 ppm	1000 ppm in the diet (50 mg/kg bw)	200	5 (as sum of β-carotene, β-apo-8'carotenal, and β-apo-8'-caroten-oic acid, ethyl, and methyl ester)	—	3 10 16

β-apo-8'-carotenoic acid, ethyl, and methyl ester	Rat	110 wk	0, 1000 ppm	1000 ppm in the diet (50 mg/kg bw)	200	5 (As sum of β-carotene, β-apo-8'-carotenal, and β-apo-8'-carotenoic acid, ethyl, and methyl ester)	—	3 10 16
Chlorophyll copper complex	Rat	2 yr	0, 1000, 10,000, 30,000 ppm (4-5% total Cu; 0.25% ionic Cu)	30,000 ppm in the diet (1500 mg/kg bw)	100	15	—	4 12 17
Chlorophyllin copper complex	Rat	2 yr	0, 1000, 10,000 30,000 ppm (4-5% total Cu; 0.25% ionic Cu)	30,000 ppm in the diet (1500 mg/kg bw)	100	15 (T) (As Na, K chlorophyllin copper complex)	—	3 4 12 17
Chocolate brown HT	Mouse	80 wk	0, 0.01%, 0.1% 0.5%	0.1% in the diet (150 mg/kg bw)	600	0.25 (T)	Brown coloration of the internal organs; increased leukocyte infiltration	12 18
Curcumin	Rat	420 day	0, 5000 ppm	5000 ppm in the diet (250 mg/kg bw) (considered to be present in turmeric at a level of 3%)	2500	0.1 (T)	—	3 19

	Species	Duration	Dose levels	No-effect level			Effects	Ref.
Erythrosine	Rat	2 yr	0, 5000, 10,000, 20,000, 50,000 ppm	5000 ppm in the diet (250 mg/kg bw)	100	2.5	Growth depression; caecal enlargement	12 4 10 20
Fast green FCF	Rat	2 yr	0, 5000, 10,000, 20,000, 50,000 ppm	50,000 ppm in the diet (2500 mg/kg bw)	200	12.5	–	4 21
Indigotine	Rat	2 yr	0, 5000, 10,000, 20,000, 50,000 ppm	10,000 ppm in the diet (500 mg/kg bw)	100	5	Growth depression	3 4 10 22
Ponceau 4R	Mouse	82 wk	0, 100, 500, 2500, 12,500 ppm	500 ppm in the diet (25 mg/kg bw)	200	0.125 (T)	Milk anemia; foamy reticulo-endothelial cells in the liver; increase incidence of glomerulonephrosis	2 3 23
Quinoline yellow	Rat	2 yr	0, 1000 ppm	1000 ppm in the diet (50 mg/kg bw)	100	0.5 (T)	–	3 4 10 24 25
Red 2G	Rat	13 wk	0, 25, 114 ppm	25 ppm in the diet (1.25 mg/kg bw)	200	0.006 (T)	Effects on spleen	12 26 27
Riboflavin	Rat	3 gen	0, 50 mg/kg bw	50 mg/kg bw	100	0.5	–	4 28

Sunset yellow FCF	Dog	7 yr	20,000 ppm	20,000 ppm in the diet (500 mg/kg bw)	100	5	—	10 29
Tartrazine	Rat	64 wk	0, 300, 3000, 15,000 ppm	15,000 ppm in the diet (750 mg/kg bw)	100	7.5	—	1 10
Turmeric	Rat	420 day	0, 5000 ppm	5000 ppm in the diet (250 mg/kg bw)	100	2.5	—	3 4 19
Yellow 2G	Rat	2 yr	0, 100, 1000, 10,000 ppm	100 ppm in the diet (5 mg/kg bw)	200	0.025 (T)	Decrease in renal concentrating ability	12 18

This table supplies a summary of the no-effect levels and other elements that have been chosen to serve as a basis for the estimation of acceptable daily intake figures (ADIs). It is important to note that this table, although inclusive for compounds evaluated in the 1978 meeting of the Joint FAO/WHO Expert Committee on Food Additives, does not stand on its own, but must be interpreted in the light of the documents referenced in column (IX) of the Table.

In assembling this Table, the following sequential steps have been adopted: (1) sorting out those food colorants for which either a numerical ADI or a temporary numerical ADI has been allocated; (2) listing them in alphabetical order in order to facilitate the location of a particular compound; (3) transcribing the no-effect level(s) as indicated in the original documents as having served as a basis for establishing ADI figures; (4) identifying the study/studies in which the no-effect level(s) has/have been demonstrated and to make reference of these studies as completely as possible; (5) construing the safety factor employed in the extrapolation process; and (6) indicating as many sources as possible that can supply additional information on the multifaceted process of toxicological and administrative decisions carried out at the international level by the Joint FAO/WHO Expert Committee on Food Additives.

REFERENCES

1. Mannell, W.A., Grice, H.C., Lu, F.C., and Allmark, M.G. Chronic toxicity. Studies on food colors. IV. Observations on the toxicity of tartrazine, amaranth and sunset yellow in rats. J. Pharm. Pharmacol., 10: 625, 1958.
2. Evaluation of certain food additives. Twenty-second report of the Joint FAO/WHO Expert Committee on Food Additives. Wld. Hlth. Org. Techn. Rep. Ser., (In press), 1978.
3. Toxicological evaluation of some food colours, enzymes, flavour enhancers, thickening agents and certain other food additives. FAO Nutrition Meetings Report Series, No. 55; WHO Food Additives Series, No. 6, 1975.
4. Toxicological evaluation of some food colours, emulsifiers, stabilizers, anti-caking agents and certain other substances. FAO Nutrition Meetings ReportSeries, No. 46A; WHO/Food Add./70.36, 1970.
5. van Esch, G.J., van Genderen, H., and Vink, H.H. Über die chronische Vetraglichkeit von Annattofarbstoff. Z. Lebensm., Untersuch. III: 93, 1959.
6. Gaunt, I.F., Farmer, M. Grasso, P., and Gangolli, S.D. Acute (mouse and rat) and short-term (rat) toxicity studies on carmoisine. Fd. Cosmet. Toxicol., 5: 179, 1967.
7. Gaunt, I.F., Farmer, M., Grasso, P., and Gangolli, S.D. Acute (mouse and rat) and short-term (rat) toxicity studies on Black PN. Fd. Cosmet. Toxicol., 5:171, 1967.
8. Gaunt, I.F., Carpanini, F.M.B., Grasso, P., and Kiss, I.S. Long-term feeding study on Black PN in rats. Fd. Cosmet. Toxicol., 10: 17, 1972.
9. Mannell, W.A., Grice, H.C., and Allmark, M.G. Chronic toxicity studies on food colours. V. Observations on the toxicity of Brilliant Blue FCF, Guinea Green B and Benzyl Violet 4B in rats. J. Pharm. Pharmacol., 14: 378, 1962.
10. Specifications for identity, purity, and toxicological evaluation of food colours. FAO Nutrition Meetings Report Series, No. 38B: WHO/Food Add./66.25, 1966.

11. Essais de toxicité avec la canthaxanthine. Unpublished report sub-
    mitted to WHO by Hoffman La Roche. Summary in Ref. 2, p. 58, 1966.
12. Evaluation of certain food additives. Twenty-first report of the
    Joint FAO/WHO Expert Committee on Food Additives. Wld. Hlth. Org.
    Techn. Rep. Ser., No. 617, 1978.
13. Summary of toxicological data on certain food additives. Document
    resulting from the Twenty-first report of the Joint FAO/WHO Expert
    Committee on Food Additives. WHO Food Additives Series, No. 12, 1978.
14. Kay, J.G. and Calandra, J.C. Subacute oral toxicity of caramel
    colourings in dogs and rats. Unpublished report from Industrial Bio-
    Test Laboratories Inc., Northbrook, Illinois, submitted by Corn
    Products Refining Co., Argo, Illinois, 1962.
15. Oser, B.L. Toxicological feeding study of "acid-proof" caramel. Un-
    published report from Food and Drug Research Laboratories Inc.,
    N.Y., submitted by D.D. Williamson & Co., Inc., Long Island City,
    N.Y., 1963.
16. Bagdon, R.E., Zbinden, G., and Studer, A. Chronic toxicity studies
    of p-carotene. Toxic. Appl. Pharmacol., 2: 225, 1960.
17. Harrison, J.W.E., Levin, S.E., and Trabin, B. The safety and fate
    of potassium sodium copper chlorophyllin and other copper compounds.
    J. Amer. Pharmacol., Sci. Ed., 43: 722, 1954.
18. Drake, J.J.P., Butterworth, K.R., Gaunt, I.F., and Hardy, J. Long-
    term toxicity studies of chocolate brown HT in mice. Unpublished re-
    port from the British Industrial Biological Research Association
    (Report No. 16/1975) Summary in Ref. 13.
19. Truhaut, R., C.R. on 18ème Congrès de la Féderation Internationale
    Pharmaceutique, Bruxelles, 8-15 September 1968. Summary in Ref. 3,
    p. 120.
20. Hansen, W.H., Zwickey, R.E., Brouwer, J.B., and Fitzhugh, O.G.
    Long-term studies on Erythrosine. I. Effects in rats and dogs. Fd.
    Cosmet. Toxicol., 11: 527, 1973.
21. Hansen, W.H., Long, E.L., Davis, K.J., Nelson, A.A., and Fitzhugh,
    O.G. Chronic toxicity of three food colourings: Guinea Green B,
    Light Green SF Yellowish, and Fast Green FCF in rats, dogs, and
    mice. Fd. Cosmet. Toxicol., 4: 389, 1966.
22. Hansen, F.H., Fitzhugh, O.G., Nelson, A.A., and Davis, K.J. Chronic
    toxicity of two food colours, Brilliant Blue FCF and Indigotine.
    Toxic. Appl. Pharmacol., 8: 29, 1966.
23. Mason, P.L., Gaunt, I.F., Butterworth, K.R., and Hardy, J. Long-
    term toxicity study of Ponceau 4R in mice. Unpublished report by
    the British Industrial Biological Association (Report 1/1974) 1974.
    Summary in Ref. 3. p. 111.
24. Oettel, H., Frohberg, H., Nothdurft, H., and Wilhelm, G. Die Prü-
    fung einiger synthetischer Farbostoffe auf ihre Eignung zur Leben-
    smittelfärbung. Arch. Toxikol., 21: 9, 1965.
25. Toxicological evaluation of some food colours, thickening agents,
    and certain other substances. FAO Nutrition Meetings Report Series,
    No. 55A; WHO Food Additives Series, No. 8, 1975.
26. Jenkins, F.P., Salmon, G., and Gellatly, J.B.M. Sub-acute toxicity
    of red 2G in sausage meat. Unpublished report from Unilever Re-
    search Laboratories. 1966. Summary in Ref. 13.
27. Gellatly, J.B.M., and Burrough, R. Toxicity of Ref. 2G. Effect of
    feeding to rats in a sausage meat diet for 90 days: pathology. Un-
    published report from Unilever Research Labs. 1968. Summary in Ref.
    13.
28. Unna, K., and Greslin, J.G. Studies on the toxicity and pharmacology
    of riboflavin. J. Pharmacol. Exp. Ther., 76: 75, 1942.

29. Summary of toxicity studies on colours (FD and C yellow No. 6). Unpublished report from the US Food and Drug Administration, 1964.
Summary in Ref. 10, p. 86.

TABLE III Toxicological Data Profiles for Food Colorants

COMPOUND	BIOCHEMICAL ASPECTS			SPECIAL TOXICOLOGICAL STUDIES								ACUTE TOXICITY								SHORT-TERM TOXICOLOGICAL STUDIES						LONG-TERM TOXICOLOGICAL STUDIES			observations in man	TOXICOLOGICAL EVALUATION NO-EFFECT LEVELS		
	absorption, distribution, and excretion	metabolism	effects on enzymes and other bio-chemical parameters	carcinogenicity	metabolites	mutagenicity	pharmacological effects	reproduction	sensitization	teratogenicity	others	cat	dog	guinea-pig	mouse	pig	rabbit	rat	other species	cat	dog	mouse	pig	rat	other species	mouse	rat	gerbil		mouse	rat	dog
Acid fuchsine FB			3	4											1						2											
Acridine orange			3 12	9 10		1 2 4 5 6 11									8						2						4					
Alkali blue															1									1	1							
Alkannin/alkanet															2			2				1										
Allura red AC	17	8 9 24		13 14 15	6	2 3 4 5 6		1 7			12 21 22 23		18					17			10 20		16 19			13 15	11 14					

Aluminium (metal)	19 20 22 31 38 40 41	20 31	14 17 20 21 23 27 28	12 13 30 33 34 35	29	25 31 32	5 10 11 18	16 31	16 37	2 32 3 4	6 38	34 24 33	1 7 8 9 10 11 15 26 36 39 40 42
							9						24 33
													2 49

| Amaranth | 25 55 59 | 53 54 55 56 58 | 1 28 32 42 46 57 60 70 | 3 6 10 11 13 16 17 24 47 50 57 68 | 22 69 30 36 44 45 51 52 | 12 | 54 | 7 8 9 11 20 39 41 48 62 | 7 14 | 7 8 9 15 19 22 23 33 34 35 37 38 40 41 43 48 61 64 65 | 16 17 18 21 26 50 63 65 69 | 4 5 | 10 | 66 27 32 67 | 24 29 6 11 21 31 47 68 |

| Annatto | | | | 4 | | 1 | | | 5 | 3 2 | 6 | |

| Anthocyanins | 2 | | | 1 3 4 5 6 7 8 9 | | | | | | | | |

TABLE III   Toxicological Data Profiles for Food Colorants

Column groups (left to right): BIOCHEMICAL ASPECTS · SPECIAL TOXICOLOGICAL STUDIES · ACUTE TOXICITY · SHORT-TERM TOXICOLOGICAL STUDIES · LONG-TERM TOXICOLOGICAL STUDIES · observations in man · TOXICOLOGICAL EVALUATION NO-EFFECT LEVELS

COMPOUND	absorption, distribution, and excretion	metabolism	effects on enzymes and other bio-chemical parameters	carcinogenicity	metabolites	mutagenicity	pharmacological effects	reproduction	sensitization	teratogenicity	others	cat	dog	guinea-pig	mouse	pig	rabbit	rat	other species	cat	dog	mouse	pig	rat	other species	mouse	rat	gerbil	observations in man	mouse	rat	dog
Auramine	4 8 17	5 22	13 16 18	2 3 8 9 10			6								1									10		3 5	5		4 7			
Azorubine				1 3 10 15		14	21	9 11	2	19 20	10				6			6 12				10	7	6 8 10		3 15						
Beet red/betanine								1																			1					
Benzyl violet 4B	6 7 12	6 12		3 4 8 11 13 16			14								15		15	9 13			1		5	2		5	3 8 10 11 13 16					
Black 7984	2	2		2 3 4				1			2 4				2			2					5	2			1 2 3					

Colorant	Numbers
Blue VRS	3	2 4 5 6 7 8 9 11 12	8 9 12	1 10	10	2	1 1 7 10	14 4 8 9 11 13 15
Brilliant black PN	9 13	6 7 11 14 16	2 3 10 15	12	1	7 8	7	7 6	4 5 9
Brilliant blue FCF	3 4 10 11 12 13 14	10 11	6 21	5 7 19	1	19	8	8	16	8 9 8	6 7 8	2 2 9 20 15 17 18 19 22
Brown FK	5 6 9	6 7 14 17 19 22 24	12 20 21 24	23	10 13 15 18	4 4 11	4 4 11	1 3 16	6 8 9 12 16	25 26	17
Butter Yellow	1	1
Canthaxanthine	1

TABLE III   Toxicological Data Profiles for Food Colorants

COMPOUND	BIOCHEMICAL ASPECTS			SPECIAL TOXICOLOGICAL STUDIES								ACUTE TOXICITY								SHORT-TERM TOXICOLOGICAL STUDIES						LONG-TERM TOXICOLOGICAL STUDIES			observations in man	TOXICOLOGICAL EVALUATION NO-EFFECT LEVELS		
	absorption, distribution, and excretion	metabolism	effects on enzymes and other bio-chemical parameters	carcinogenicity	metabolites	mutagenicity	pharmacological effects	reproduction	sensitization	teratogenicity	others	cat	dog	guinea-pig	mouse	pig	rabbit	rat	other species	cat	dog	mouse	pig	rat	other species	mouse	rat	gerbil		mouse	rat	dog
Caramel	14				5 11 16 17 18 20 21 27 28 40 41	6		1 4 39		1 24 25								7 8 10				31		3 7 8 10 12 13 15 19 26 29 30 32 33 34 35 36 38			1 4 9 37		2 22 23			
Carbon blacks	16	1 10 11 12 13 15 17		4 9 14 16 18 20 21							2 8																		3 5 6 7 19 23			

Name	Reference numbers
Carotenal, β-apo-8	4, 5 · 3 · 6, 7, 8, 9, 10 · 2 · 3 · 1 · 9
Carotene, β synthetic	3, 5, 6, 8, 10, 12, 13 · 1, 4, 7, 11 · 2, 13 · 1
Carotenoic acid, β-apo-8	3, 4 · 2 · 2 · 1
Cartja,is	1 · 3 · 5 · 3 · 1, 2
Chlorophylls, chlorophyll, Cu complex, chlorophyllin, Cu complex	1, 3, 4 · 2 · 3 · 8, 8, 8, 8 · 8, 8 · 7 · 6
Chocolate brown FB	2, 6 · 2 · 5 · 5 · 1, 5, 6 · 3, 4
Chocolate Brown HT	4 · 6 · 7 · 7 · 5, 2 · 3, 1
Chrysoidine	6, 7, 10, 11 · 1, 2, 4, 5, 8 · 9 · 1, 2, 3, 5 · 8
Chrysoine S	4 · 5 · 3 · 1 · 6 · 2 · 5

TABLE III Toxicological Data Profiles for Food Colorants

COMPOUND	BIOCHEM: absorption, distribution, and excretion	BIOCHEM: metabolism	BIOCHEM: effects on enzymes and other bio-chemical parameters	SPECIAL: carcinogenicity	SPECIAL: metabolites	SPECIAL: mutagenicity	SPECIAL: pharmacological effects	SPECIAL: reproduction	SPECIAL: sensitization	SPECIAL: teratogenicity	SPECIAL: others	ACUTE: cat	ACUTE: dog	ACUTE: guinea-pig	ACUTE: mouse	ACUTE: pig	ACUTE: rabbit	ACUTE: rat	ACUTE: other species	SHORT-TERM: cat	SHORT-TERM: dog	SHORT-TERM: mouse	SHORT-TERM: pig	SHORT-TERM: rat	SHORT-TERM: other species	LONG-TERM: mouse	LONG-TERM: rat	LONG-TERM: gerbil	observations in man	NO-EFFECT: mouse	NO-EFFECT: rat	NO-EFFECT: dog
Chrysoine SGX "specially pure"				1, 4											1					3						1	1, 2					
Citranaxanthin					1, 5		3, 8				9		4		9			9			6			2, 10			1, 5					
Citrus red 2	4	4, 5		1, 2, 3, 6											3						3	1				2, 6	2, 3					
Cochineal/carmine/carminic acid						1, 2, 5, 6				3, 10	8, 9, 10, 11				4			3	3, 3			4		7, 12								
Congo red										1		3			4		3, 5	3	3		6, 2											
Eosin, eosin, disodium salt	10, 18	18	12, 14, 15	4, 5, 6, 9, 16, 17		11, 13									7			2				17		1			9, 17		3, 8			

Erythrosine	7 33	3 7 19 23 33	1 8 9 11 26 27 28 30 31	12 24 29 32	21 22	13 15	2 14	24		3	10	3 10 17 20 31	6	17 29	4	5	4 11 12	16 17 29 34	6	1 3 18 24 25 30 32
Fast green FCF	5 6 7 9	5 7 12	13	1 2 3 4 8 11 14	12			11			10			4	4		3 4 8		4 11 14	
Fast red E	7	3		7	6	2		(1)			5		4						7 5	
Fast yellow AB	7 11 12	6 7 12 13	2 9 14		10	1					3 5		4		15	5 8			5	
Ferrous gluconate	(2) (3) (4)								5 1 1 5	1 5									
Fluorescein	4 7	4		6	5						2 2			6		1 3			6	
Food green S	2 3	2									4			1		1 5 6				

TABLE III Toxicological Data Profiles for Food Colorants

COMPOUND	BIOCHEMICAL ASPECTS			SPECIAL TOXICOLOGICAL STUDIES								ACUTE TOXICITY								SHORT-TERM TOXICOLOGICAL STUDIES						LONG-TERM TOXICOLOGICAL STUDIES			observations in man	TOXICOLOGICAL EVALUATION NO-EFFECT LEVELS		
	absorption, distribution, and excretion	metabolism	effects on enzymes and other bio-chemical parameters	carcinogenicity	metabolites	mutagenicity	pharmacological effects	reproduction	sensitization	teratogenicity	others	cat	dog	guinea-pig	mouse	pig	rabbit	rat	other species	cat	dog	mouse	pig	rat	other species	mouse	rat	gerbil		mouse	rat	dog
Gold	1 2 4 5 6	3 6																											7			
Guinea green B	3 4 5 6 10	3 4 5 10	1	2 9 11							11							7			2	2		1		2	2 8 9 11 12					
Indanthrene blue RS				5 6					1									3						2			4 6					
Indigotine	7	9	4 8 13	1	11				14	2	15				1			1 10			5		3	4		5 6 12	5 5					

Dye	1	2	3	4	5	6	7	8	9	10	11	12	13	14	15
Light green SF	6 9 10 11 14 15 19	6 10 11 19	16 17 22 23	1 2 3 4 5 8 12 13 20 21 24 25						5	18	5 7 7	4 5 7 8 12 20 21 24	7 25	1 7 13 20
Lithol rubine BK				7		8	6	3	2	5	1		7	5	
Lycopene	1												1		
Magenta				1 3 5 6 8	1	6							3 9	5 8	2 4 7
Malachite green			5 6 7	1						4	8 9		2 3 8 9	1	
Methanil yellow				1	3					2		1	3		
Methyl violet				2	2					1	1		3		
Naphthol blue black	1									3			1		
Naphthol yellow			1	4						3		4	2 3	3	
Nigrosine				1 3						2	2	2		3	1 2

TABLE III Toxicological Data Profiles for Food Colorants

COMPOUND	BIOCHEMICAL ASPECTS			SPECIAL TOXICOLOGICAL STUDIES								ACUTE TOXICITY								SHORT-TERM TOXICOLOGICAL STUDIES						LONG-TERM TOXICOLOGICAL STUDIES			observations in man	TOXICOLOGICAL EVALUATION NO-EFFECT LEVELS		
	absorption, distribution, and excretion	metabolism	effects on enzymes and other bio-chemical parameters	carcinogenicity	metabolites	mutagenicity	pharmacological effects	reproduction	sensitization	teratogenicity	others	cat	dog	guinea-pig	mouse	pig	rabbit	rat	other species	cat	dog	mouse	pig	rat	other species	mouse	rat	gerbil		mouse	rat	dog
Oil orange SS	10	4, 5, 11, 12	13	1, 5, 6, 7, 10, 13	1, 6, 11		11, 12						8				8	8			2, 9			2, 3, 5, 8, 10, 13	2, 8	2, 6	1, 9, 10, 13		4			
Oil Orange XO				1, 4, 6, 9, 15	1, 11		12, 14											5			2, 7	2, 5		2, 5, 8, 9, 15	2, 5	2, 4, 6	1, 7, 15		3			
Oil yellow AB		10, 12	11	1, 5, 7, 9, 13, 15			10, 14								2, 12						6, 8	6, 7		1, 2, 7, 8, 9, 13, 15	1, 2, 5	3, 7	1, 5, 6, 7, 9, 13		4			

	1	2	3	4	5	6	7	8	9	10	11	12
Oil yellow OB	11	8, 9	10	1, 5, 15	8, 14		2, 11	4, 5, 6	1, 5, 6, 7, 12, 15	2, 3, 5	4, 5	13
Oleoresin of paprika	1, 3, 4, 6, 7, 8	13, 14	8, 12	2	5	1, 4	2		2	1		
Orange I	14, 16	4, 5, 6, 10, 11	9	5, 7, 11	6, 13, 16	1	1, 2	15, 1, 5, 15	3, 5, 16	7, 3, 5, 9, 11	1, 3, 4	
Orange II		3, 4		1	2	4				1		
Orange G	4, 6, 12	2, 3, 5, 10	9	3, 13		1				1, 3, 13		12
Orange GGN	6, 8	2, 3, 5, 10	7	4, 5, 13	1		4	4, 11	9	12, 3, 4, 5, 12		
Orange RN	2	2, 6, 7, 10, 11, 13	13	12	1		1	12	4, 5, 8, 9	1, 1, 12		
Orchil/orcein									1	1		

TABLE III   Toxicological Data Profiles for Food Colorants

COMPOUND	BIOCHEMICAL ASPECTS — absorption, distribution, and excretion	metabolism	effects on enzymes and other bio-chemical parameters	SPECIAL TOXICOLOGICAL STUDIES — carcinogenicity	metabolites	mutagenicity	pharmacological effects	reproduction	sensitization	teratogenicity	others	ACUTE TOXICITY — cat	dog	guinea-pig	mouse	pig	rabbit	rat	other species	SHORT-TERM TOXICOLOGICAL STUDIES — cat	dog	mouse	pig	rat	other species	LONG-TERM TOXICOLOGICAL STUDIES — mouse	rat	gerbil	observations in man	TOXICOLOGICAL EVALUATION NO-EFFECT LEVELS — mouse	rat	dog
Patent blue V	4	4, 8, 12, 16	3	1, 2, 3	1							5			5			5	5					1, 3			5					
Ponceau 2R	4, 8, 14, 16	4, 8, 12, 16	12, 15	1, 2, 6, 9, 10, 11, 17, 18	1										7			7						7		1, 2, 9, 11, 17	3, 6, 9, 10, 18					
Ponceau 3R	5, 19	5, 11, 12, 13, 14, 15	6, 18	1, 4, 7, 8, 9, 10, 16, 17, 20	2							19			19			19		19	8	4		6, 7		8	1, 8, 10, 16, 19, 20		3			

Dye											
Ponceau 4R	17	17 20	17 18 19 21	1 2	16 4 5 15 12 13	6	6 9	8	7 6 10	14 1 9	3
Ponceau 6R			3	2	5 1		4	3	7 4	4	6
Ponceau SX	5 8 9 10 11	4		1 7 3 13	7 12	6		2 3	4	3 2 3 13	
Quercitin/quercitron	8 11	2 7 8 10	2	3 5 4 6		1			9	1	
Quinoline yellow	2 4		7	6	9 3 8	5	1		4 7	2 7	
Red 10B	2 4	2				1 1 2	1 1 2		1 3		
Red 2G	4 21 3 4 12 16 22	15	5 6 8 9 10	18 19 20	7 1 1 2		11 13		14 17		
Resorcine brown									1		
Rhodamine B	9 10 11 9 10 11	7	2 3 4 12 2 6 5		11	8	1 4 11		2 8 12		
Rhodamine GG			1 3 1 2	1		3		3			

TABLE III Toxicological Data Profiles for Food Colorants

COMPOUND	BIOCHEMICAL ASPECTS — absorption, distribution, and excretion	metabolism	effects on enzymes and other biochemical parameters	SPECIAL TOXICOLOGICAL STUDIES — carcinogenicity	metabolites	mutagenicity	pharmacological effects	reproduction	sensitization	teratogenicity	others	ACUTE TOXICITY — cat	dog	guinea-pig	mouse	pig	rabbit	rat	other species	SHORT-TERM TOXICOLOGICAL STUDIES — cat	dog	mouse	pig	rat	other species	LONG-TERM TOXICOLOGICAL STUDIES — mouse	rat	gerbil	observations in man	TOXICOLOGICAL EVALUATION NO-EFFECT LEVELS — mouse	rat	dog
Riboflavin	2, 3, 4, 7, 9	6						1, 8						10					5, 10			10			10								
Saffron/Crocin crocitin						3				2	2				1														2, 3			
Scarlet GN	4		5			3			1						2			2			2		6	2			2					
Silver	1, 2, 7, 11, 16, 25	7	5, 6, 8, 13, 19, 25, 28, 30	21		20	9, 14, 22	15			29		25								25			4, 10	4, 18, 23		17		3, 12, 24, 27			

Sudan I	9	4 5 9	3 4 5 11	1 2 3 6 7 8 10 11			13 13		1 2 3 6 7 8	12	11 10	
Sudan III	7	2 7		9 10 12 13			2	2	1 2 6 8 13		9 12 / 10	
Sudan IV	8 11	8 11		2 3 4 5 6 7 9 10 12 13 14 16 17					2 3 4 6 7 9 10 17	15	12 5 / 13 14 16	1
Sudan G	5	5		2 3			1	4	1 3		6 2 / 4	
Sudan red G		2		2			1	3	1		2	
Sunset yellow FCF	5 6 20 23	5 14 20 21 22	11 13 19 24 25	1 4 7 10 12 18 28	1 4 16 26	2 19	8	8 15 17	1 4 9	9 8 11 27	1 1 10 18 19 28	3

TABLE III Toxicological Data Profiles for Food Colorants

COMPOUND	BIOCHEMICAL ASPECTS			SPECIAL TOXICOLOGICAL STUDIES								ACUTE TOXICITY								SHORT-TERM TOXICOLOGICAL STUDIES						LONG-TERM TOXICOLOGICAL STUDIES			observations in man	TOXICOLOGICAL EVALUATION NO-EFFECT LEVELS		
	absorption, distribution, and excretion	metabolism	effects on enzymes and other bio-chemical parameters	carcinogenicity	metabolites	mutagenicity	pharmacological effects	reproduction	sensitization	teratogenicity	others	cat	dog	guinea-pig	mouse	pig	rabbit	rat	other species	cat	dog	mouse	pig	rat	other species	mouse	rat	gerbil	observations in man	mouse	rat	dog
Tartrazine	4 5 6 8 15 20 21	1 5 15 19 27 28	9 10 14 22 23	17 18		16		24	3	24	18				2			11			7 11			10 13		12 17 25 26	7 11					
Thiazine brown R															2			2		1							2					
Titanium dioxide	1 2 5 7		3 4 6			1	4	5										2						1 7								
Turmeric/curcumin			3			1					2													5	5	5	6					
Ultramarines								8		10					11 12		11	7	1 5						6				2 3 4			

Violamine R			1		1	1
Violet 5 BN						1
Water blue I			1		1	
Xanthophyls	1					
Yellow 2G	6			3	4	2 5
	7					
	8					
	1					
	6					
	9					
	10					
	11					
	12					
Yellow 27175 N	1	2	2	2	2	2

REFERENCES

ACID FUCHSINE FB

1. Hecht. G. Unpublished results. In: Deutsche Forschunsgemeinschaft, Farbstoff-Kommission, Toxikologische Daten von Farbstoffen, und ihre Zulassung fur Lebensmittel in verschiedenen Landen, Mitt.6 (2), Wiesbaden, Steiner Verlag, p. 81, 1957.
2. Kreb, H.A. and Wittgenstein, A. Disappearance of intravenously injected dyes from blood plasma. Klin. Wchnschr. 5: 320, 1926.
3. Sikorska, E. and Krauze, S. Suppressing effects of some food color and cosmetic dyes on the activity of succinic oxidase. Roczniki Panstwowego Zakladu Hig. 13: 457-66, 1962.
4. Willheim, R. and Ivy, A.C. A preliminary study concerning the possibility of dietary carcinogenesis. Gastroenterology. 23: 1-19, 1953.

ACRIDINE ORANGE

1. Davies, P.J., Evans, W.E., and Parry, J.M. Mitotic recombination induced by chemical and physical agents in the yeast Saccharomyces cerevisiae. Mutation Res., 29: 301-14, 1975.
2. Fahrig, R. Acridine-induced mitotic gene conversion (paramutation) in Saccharomyces cerevisiae: the effect of two different modes of binding to DNA. Mutation Res. 10: 509-14, 1970.
3. Lerman, L.S. The structure of the DNA-acridine complex. Proc. Nat. Acad. Sci. (Wash.), 49: 94-102, 1963.
4. McCann, J., Choi, E., Yamasaki, E., and Ames, B.N. Detection of carcinogens as mutagens in the Salmonella/microsome test: assay of 300 chemicals. Proc. Nat. Acad. Sci. (Wash.), 72: 5135-5139, 1975.
5. Nakai, S. and Saeki, T. Induction of mutation by photodynamic action in Escherichia coli. Genet. Res. (Camb.), 5: 158-161, 1964.
6. Orgel, A. and Brenner, S. Mutagenesis of bacteriophage T4 by acridines. J. Molec. Biol. 3: 762-68, 1961.
7. Rosenkranz, H.S. and Carr, H.S. Possible hazard in use of gentian violet. Brit. Med. J., iii, 702-703, 1971.
8. Rubbo, S.D. The influence of chemical constitution on toxicity. I. A general survey of the acridine series. Brit. J. Exp. Path., 28: 1-11, 1947.
9. Trainin, N., Kaye, A.M., and Berenblum, I. Influence of mutagens on the initiation of skin carcinogenesis. Biochem. Pharmacol. 13: 263-67, 1964.
10. Van Duuren, B.L., Sivak, A., Katz, C., and Melchionne, S. Tumorigenicity of acridine orange. Brit. J. Cancer, 23: 587-90, 1969.
11. Zampieri, A. and Greenberg, J. Mutagenesis by acridine orange and proflavine in Escherichia coli strain S. Mutation Res., 2:552-556, 1965.
12. Zelenin, A.V. and Liapunova, E.A. Inhibition of protein synthesis by acridine orange. Nature (London), 204: 45-6, 1964.

ALKALI BLUE

1. Farbwerke Hoechst, A.G. Unpublished Report, October 1964.

ALKANET/ALKANNIN

1. Majláthová, L. Feeding trial with alkannin in mice. Nahrung, 15: 505-508, 1971.
2. Majláthová, L. and Szokolay, A. Acute toxicity of the food additive alkannin. Cs. hygiena VI, 2-3: 132-135, 1961.

ALLURA RED AC

1. Blackmore, R.H., Olson, W.A., and Voelker, R.W. Two-generation reproduction study in rats with Red Z-4576. Unpublished report from the Hazleton Labs., Inc. Falls Church, Va. to Allied Chemical Corp., Morriston, N.J., U.S.A., 1969. Summary in: WHO/FAO 1975b, pp. 38-39.
2. Guyton, C.L. and Reno, F.E. Metabolic disposition of ^{35}S allura red in the dog and rat (FD and C Red, No. 40). Final report. Unpublished report from Hazleton Labs. America, Inc. to Allied Chem. Corp., Morriston, N.J., U.S.A. 1975.
3. Guyton, C.L. and Stanovick, R.P., Determination of the metabolites of allura red AC in the rat and dog. Final report. Unpublished report from Hazleton Labs. America, Inc. to Allied Chem. Corp. Morriston, N.J., 1975.
4. Metabolites of Red No. 40. Mutagenicity investigations on cresidine sulfonic acid and the amino Schaeffer's acid in the Ames plates. FDA's Labs. Interim report of the Working Group on FD and C Red, No. 40, January 19, 1977.
5. Mutagenicity investigations with allura red. Heritable transloca-tion. Stanford Research Institute. Interim report of the Working Group on FD and C Red, No. 40, January 19, 1977.
6. Mutagenicity investigations with allura red. Saccharomyces cere-visiae. Genetic Toxicology Branch of the FDA. Interim report of the Working Group on FD and C Red No. 40, January 19, 1977.
7. Mutagenicity investigations with allura red. Salmonella typhimurium. Genetic Toxicology Branch of the FDA. Interim report of the Working Group on FD and C Red No. 40, January 19, 1977.
8. Mutagenicity investigations with allura red. Sex-linked recessive lethals. Drosophila melanogaster. Bowling Green University, Ohio, USA. Interim report of the Working Group on FD and C Red, No. 40, January 19, 1977.
9. Olson, W.A. and Voelker, R.W. 104-week dietary administration to dogs of Red Z-4576. Unpublished report from Hazleton Labs., Inc. Falls Church, Va., submitted to Allied Chem. Corp., Morriston, N.J., 1970. Summary in: WHO/FAO 1975b, p. 40.
10. Olson, W.A. and Voelker, R.W., 21-month dietary administration to albino rats of Red Z-4576. Unpublished report from Hazleton Labs., Inc., Falls Church, Va., submitted to Allied Chem. Corp., Morriston, N.J., 1970. Summary in: WHO/FAO 1975b, pp. 40-41.
11. Reno, F.E. Teratology study in rabbits. FD and C 40. Unpublished report from Hazleton Labs., Inc., Falls Church, Va., submitted to Allied Chemical Corp., Morriston, N.J., 1974. Summary in: WHO/FAO 1975b, p. 39.
12. Reno, F.E. Combined carcinogenic bioassay and lifetime dietary ad-ministration—mice. Unpublished report from Hazleton Labs., Inc. submitted to Allied Chem. Corp., Morriston, N.J. 1974.
13. Reno, F.E. Combined carcinogenic bioassay and two-year dietary ad-ministration—rats. Unpublished report from Hazleton Labs., Inc. submitted to Allied Chem. Corp., Morriston, N.J., 1974.

14. Reno, F.E. Combined carcinogenic bioassay and lifetime dietary administration in mice (second mice study). Unpublished report from hazleton Labs., Inc. submitted to Allied Chem. Corp., Morriston, N.J., 1976.

15. Reproduction study with allura red (rat). Unpublished report from the US Food and Drug Administration, 1974, p. 39.

16. Sondergaard, D., Hansen, E.V. and Würtzen, G. A short-term study in the pig of the effects on the liver and on the blood of eight azo dyes. Toxicology, 8: 381-86, 1977.

17. Weir, R.J. Acute oral administration to rats of five experimental nontoxic red colours. Unpublished report from Hazleton Labs., Inc., Falls Church, Va., submitted to Allied Chem. Corp., Morriston, N.J., 1965. Summary in: WHO-FAO 1975b, pp. 38-39.

18. Weir, R.J. Acute oral toxicity—Dogs. Five experimental nontoxic red colours. Unpublished report from Hazleton Labs., Inc., Falls Church, Va., submitted to Allied Chem. Corp., Morriston, N.J., 1965. Summary in: WHO/FAO 1975b, p. 39.

19. Weir, R.J. Six-week dietary feeding study in rats with experimental nontoxic Red Z-4576, Red Z-4578, Red Z-4598, and Red Z-4808. Unpublished report from Hazleton Labs., Inc., Falls Church, Va. Submitted to Allied Chem. Corp., Morriston, N.J. 1966. Summary in: WHO/FAO 1975b, p.40.

20. Weir, R.J. Six-week oral administration to dogs of experimental nontoxic Reds Z-4576, Z-4578, Z-4598, and Z-4808. Unpublished report from Hazleton Labs., Inc., Falls Church, Va., submitted to Allied Chem. Corp., Morriston, N.J. 1966. Summary in: WHO/FAO 1975b, p. 40.

21. Weir, R.J. Acute dermal application to rabbits of Red Z-4576. Unpublished report from Hazleton Labs., Inc., Falls Church, Va., submitted to Allied Chem. Corp., Morriston, N.J., 1967. Summary in: WEO/FAO 1975b, p. 39.

22. Weir, R.J. Repeated dermal application study in rabbits. Nontoxic Red Z-4576. Unpublished report from Hazleton Labs., Inc., Falls Church, Va., submitted to Allied Chem. Corp., Morriston, N.J., 1968. Summary in: WHO/FAO 1975b, p. 39.

23. Weir, R.J. Repeated dermal application to Swiss mice of Red Z-4576. Unpublished report from Hazleton Labs., Inc., Falls Church, Va., submitted to Allied Chem. Corp., Morriston, N.J., 1970. Summary in: WHO/FAO 1975b, p. 40.

24. White, R.G. Metabolic fate of orally ingested nontoxic Red Z-4576. Unpublished report from Hazleton Labs., Inc., Falls Church, Va., submitted to Allied Chem. Corp., Morriston, N.J., 1970. Summary in: WHO/FAO 1975b, p. 38.

ALUMINUM (metal)

1. A short-term study in the dog. Unpublished report (IBT No. B747) from Industrial Bio-Test Labs submitted to Stauffer Chemical Company, 1972. Summary in WHO/FAO 1978 (In press).

2. A short-term study in the dog. Unpublished report (IBT No. B747) from Industrial Bio-Test Labs sumbitted to Stauffer Chemical Company, 1972a. Summary in WHO/FAO 1978 (In press).

3. A short-term study in the dog. Unpublished report (IBT No. B747) from Industrial Bio-Test Labs submitted to Stauffer Chemical Company, 1972b. Summary in WEO/FAO 1978 (In press).

4. Alfrey, A.C., Le Gendre, G.R., and Kaehney, W.D. The dialysis encephalopathy syndrome: possible aluminum intoxication. New. Engl. J. Med., 294(4): 184-185, 1976.

5. Bennett, R.W., Persaud, T.V.N., and Moore, K.L. Teratological studies with aluminum in the rat. Teratology, 9(3): A-14, 1974.
6. Berlyne, G.M., Ben-Ari, J., Knopf, E., Yagil, R., Weinberger, G., and Danovitch, G.M. Aluminium toxicity in rats. Lancet, 1:564, 1972.
7. Berlyne, G.M., Ben-Ari, J., Pest, D., Weiberger, J., Stern, M., Gilmore, G.R., Livine, R.,Hyperaluminemia from aluminum resins in renal failure. Lancet, 1: 494, 1970.
8. Clarkson, E.M., Luck, V.A., Hyson, W.V., Baily, R.R., Eastwood, J.B., Woodhead, J.S., Clements, V.R., O'Riordan, J.L.H., De Wardener, H.E. The effect of aluminium hydroxide on calcium, phosphorus and aluminium balances, the serum parathyroid hormone concentration, and the aluminium content of bone in patients with chronic renal failure. Clin. Sci., 43: 519-531, 1972.
9. Crapper, D.R., Krishnan, S.S., and Dalton, A.J. Brain aluminium distributions in Alzheimer's disease and experimental neurofibrillary degeneration, Science, 180: 511-513, 1973.
10. Crapper, D.R., Krishnan, S.S., and Quittkat, S. Aluminium neurofibrillary degeneration and Alzheimer's disease. Brain Res., 99: 67-80, 1976.
11. Crapper, D.R., and Tomko, G.J. Neuronal correlates of an encephalopathy induced by aluminium neurofibrillary degeneration. Brain Res., 97: 253-64, 1975.
12. Furst, A. Trace elements related to specific chronic disease: cancer. Geol. Soc. Amer. Mem., 123: 109, 1971.
13. Furst, A. and Haro, R.T. A survey of metal carcinogenesis. Progr. Exp. Tumor Res., 12: 102, 1969.
14. Gisselbrecht, H., Baufle, G.H. and Duvernoy, H. Annal. Scient. Univ. Besancon Med., 44: 29, 1957.
15. Hamilton, 1972 (see silver, Ref. 12).
16. Hart, M.M. and Adamson, R.H. Antitumour activity and toxicity of salts of inorganic group IIIa metals: aluminium, gallium, and thallium. Proc. Nat. Acad. Sci., 68:1923-1926, 1971.
17. Isaac, O. and Ferch, H. Uber das physiologische Verhalten von hochdispersen Oxides des Siliciums. Aluminiums and Titans. Dtsch. Apoth. Ztg., 116: 1867, 1976.
18. King, G.A., De Boni, U., and Crapper, D.R. Effect of aluminium upon conditioned avoidance response acquisition in the absence of neurofibrillary degeneration. Pharm. Biochem. and Behav., 3: 1003-1009, 1975.
19. Kirsher, J.B. J. Clin. Invest. 22: 47, 1943.
20. Kortus, J. The carbohydrate metabolism accompanying intoxication by aluminium in the rat. Experientia, 23: 912-913, 1967.
21. Kratchovil, B., Boyer, S.L., and Hicks, G.P. Effects of metals on the activation and inhibition of isocitric dehydrogenase. Anal. Chem., 39: 45, 1967.
22. Jones, J.H. Metabolism of calcium and phosphorus as influenced by addition to diet of salts of metals which form insoluble phosphates. Am. J. Physiol., 124: 230-237, 1938.
23. Langenback, W., and Schellenberger, A. Uber die decarboxylierung der Benztraubensaure durch Aluminium-ionen. Arch. Biochem. Biophys. 69: 22, 1957.
24. Lyman, J.F. and Scott, E. Effects of the injection of tartrate or sodium aluminium sulfate baking powders upon growth, reproduction and kidney structure in the rat. Am. J. Hyg., 12: 271-282, 1930.
25. Mackenzie, K. Biochemistry of aluminium; effect of aluminium on growth and reproduction in the rat; occurrence of aluminium in the

thyroid; intestinal absorption of aluminium in the rabbit. Biochem. J., 26: 833-834, 1932.

26. McLaughin, A.I.G., Kazantzis, G., King, E., Teare, D., Porter, R.J., and Owen, R. Pulmonary fibrosis and encephalopathy associated with the inhalation of aluminium dust. Brit. J. Ind. Med., 19: 253-263, 1962.

27. Meredith, P.A., Moore, M.R., and Goldberg, A. The effect of aluminium, lead, and zinc on gamma-aminolaevulonic acid dehydratase. Biochem. Soc. Trans., 2: 1243-1245, 1974.

28. Nathanson, J.A., and Bloom, F.E. Heavy metals and adenosine cyclic 3',5'-monophosphate metabolism possible relevance to heavy metal toxicity. Mol. Pharm. 12: 390-398, 1976.

29. Nishioka, 1975 (see silver Ref. 20).

30. O'Gara, R.W., and Brown, J.M., Comparison, of the carcinogenic actions of subcutaneous implants of iron and aluminum in rodents. J. Nat. Cancer Inst., 38: 947-953, 1967.

31. Ondreicka, R., Grinter, E., and Kortus, J. Chronic toxicity of aluminum in rats and mice and its effects on phosphorus metabolism. Brit. J. Ind. Med., 23: 305-311, 1966.

32. Schaeffer, G., Fontes, G., LeBreton, E., Oberling, E., and Thivolle, L. The dangers of certain mineral baking-powders based on alum, when used for human nutrition. J. Hyg., 28: 92-99, 1928.

33. Schroeder, M.A., and Mitchener, M. Life-time studies in rats of aluminum, beryllium, and tungsten. J. Nutr., 105: 421-427, 1975.

34. Schroeder, M.A., and Mitchener, M. Life-time effects of mercury, methylmercury, and nine other metals on mice. J. Nutr., 105: 452-458, 1975.

35. Shubik and Hartwell, 1969 (see butter yellow).

36. Sorenson, J.R.J., Campbell, I.R., Tepper, L.B., and Ling, R.D. Aluminum in the environment and human health. Environm. Health. Persp., 8: 3-95, 1974.

37. Spector, W.S. Handbook of toxicology, Vol. I. Acute toxicities. Philadelphia. Saunders Ed., Par 16, 1956.

38. Thurston, H., Gimore, G.R., and Swales, J.P. Aluminum retention and toxicity in chronic renal failure. Lancet I, 881-885, 1972.

39. Tipton, I.H., and Cook, M.J. Trace elements in human tissues. III. Subjects from Africa, the Near and Far East, and Europe, Health Phys., 11: 403, 1965.

40. Tipton, I.H., Stewart, P.L., and Martin, P.C. Trace elements in diets and excreta. Health Phys., 1683-1689, 1966.

41. Underhill, F.P., Peterman, F.I., and Sperandeo. Studies in metabolism of aluminum; note on toxic effects produced by subcutaneous injection of aluminum salts. Am. J. Physiol. 90: 76-82, 1929.

42. Verberckmoes, R. Aluminum toxicity in rats. Lancet I, 750, 1972.

AMARANTH

1. Albrecht, R., Manchon, Ph., Keko-Pinto, C., and Lowy, R. Evoluation, au cours de temps, de quelques effets du Bordeaux S et du Jaune de Beurre sur l'organisme du rat. Fd. Cosm. Toxicol. 11: 175-84, 1973.

2. Amaranth: acute toxicity in the mouse. Unpublished report from the Food and Drug Administration U.S.A., 1952. Summary in: WHO/FAO 1975a, p. 16.

3. Amaranth: acute toxicity in the mouse. Unpublished report from the Food and Drug Administration U.S.A., 1959. Summary in: WHO/FAO 1975a, p. 16.

4. Amos, H.E., and Drake, J.J.P. Food additives and hypersensitivity. Int. Flav. Fd. Add. 8(1): 19-23, 1977.

5. Andrianova, M.M. Carcinogenous properties of red food pigments: amaranth, SX purple, and 4R purple, Vop. Pitan., 29: 61-65, 1970.

6. Arnold, D.W., Kennedy, Jr., GlL., Keplinger, M.L., and Calandra, J.C. Failure of FD and C Red No. 2 to produce dominant lethal effects in the mouse. Fd Cosmet. Toxicol. 14: 163-165, 1976.

7. Baigusheva, M.M. Carcinogenic properties of the amaranth paste. Vop. Pitan., 27: 46-50, 1968.

8. Bär, F., and Griepentrog, F. Die Allergenwirkung von Fremden Stoffen in den Lebensmitteln. Med. U. Ernaehr, 1: 99-104, 1960.

9. Burnett, C.M., Agersborg, H.P.K., Jr., Borzelleca, J.F., Eagle, E., Ebert, A.G., Pierce, F.C., Kirshman, J.C., and Scala, R.A. Teratogenic studies with certified colors in rats. Toxicol. Appl. Pharmacol., 29: 121, Abstract 118, 1974.

10. Carson, S. The safety evaluation of FD and C Red 2 by dermal application to rabbits. Unpublished report from the Food and Drug Research Labs, Inc. to the Toilet Goods Association, Inc. and the U.S. Food and Drug Administration, 1962. Summary in WHO/FAO 1975a, p. 16.

11. Carson, S. Skin painting studies in mice. Unpublished report from the Food and Drug Research Labs, Inc. (Lab. Rep. No 81998, 1963 study plus addendum) to the Toilet Goods Association, Inc. and to the U.S. Food and Drug Administration, 1966. Summary in WHO/FAO 1975a, p. 17.

12. Collins, T.F.X., Black, T.N., and Ruggles, D.I. Long-term effects of dietary amaranth in rats. II. Effects on fetal development. Toxicology, 3: 129-140, 1975.

13. Colins, T.F.X., Black, T.N., Ruggles, D.I., and Gray, G.C. Teratological evaluation of FD and C Red No. 2. A collaborative government-industry study. II. FDA study. J. Toxicol. Envir. Hlth. 1: 857, 1976.

14. Collins, T.F.X., Keeler, H.V., Black, T.N., and Ruggles, D.I. Long-term effects of dietary amaranth in rats, I. Effects on reproduction. Toxicology, 3: 115-128, 1975.

15. Collins, T.F.X., McLaughlin, J.C and Gray, G.C. Teratology studies on food colourings. Part I. Embryotoxicity of amaranth (FD and C Red 2) in rats. Fd. Cosmet. Toxicol., 19: 619-624, 1972.

16. Collins, T.F.X., McLaughlin, J., and Gray, G.C. Teratology studies on food colourings. Part II. Embryotoxicity of R salt and metabolites of amaranth (FD and C Red 2) in rats. Fd. Cosmet. Toxciol., II: 3 5-365, 1973.

17. Collins, T.F.X., Ruggles, D.I., Holson, Jr., J.F., Schumacher, H., Gaylor, D.W., and Kennedy, Jr., G L. Teratological evaluation of FD and C Red No. 2. A collaborative government-industry study. I. Introduction, Experimental materials and procedures. J. Toxicol. Environ. Hlth., 1: 851, 1976.

18. Cook, J.W., Hewett, C.L., Kennaway, E.L., and Kennaway, N.M. Effects produced in the livers of mice by azonaphthalenes and related compounds. Amer. J. Cancer, 40: 62-77, 1940.

19. Despopoulos, A. Renal and hepatic transport of food dyes, J. Pharmac. Exper. Therap., 163: 222-228, 1968.

20. Ershoff, B.H. Protective effects of cholestyramine in rats fed a low-fiber diet containing toxic doses of sodium cyclamate and amaranth. Proc. Soc. Exp. Biol. Med., 152: 253-256, 1976.

21. Ershoff, B.H., and Thurston, E.W. Effects of diet on amarnath (FD and C Red No. 2). Toxicity in the rat J. Nutr., 104: 937-942.

22. Galea, V., Ariesan, M., and Luputiu, G. Biochemical alteration in the liver of white rats under the influence of synthetic organic dyes, orange GGN and amaranth. Farmacia (Bucharest), 10: 531-533, 1962.

23. Galea, V., Preda, N., Popa, L., Sendrea, D., and Simu, G. Recherches toxicologiques sur le colorant amaranthe. J. Europ. Toxicol., 5: 167-173, 1972.

24. Garner, R.C., and Nutman, C.A. Testing of some azo dyes and their reduction products for mutagenicity using S. typhimurium (TA 1538). Mutat. Res., 44: 9-19, 1977.

25. Gordon, L.A., and Taylor, J.M. Chronic feeding study of amaranth in rats. Unpublished report submitted by the U.S. Food and Drug Adm. to WHO, 1975. Summary in WHO/FAO 1978 (to be issued).

26. Graham, R.C.B., and Allmark, M.G. Screening of some food colors for estrogenic activity. Toxicol. Appl. Pharmacol., 1: 144-146.

27. Haley, S., Plank, J.B., Wright, P.L., and Keplinger, M.L. Teratogenic study with FD and C Red No. 2 in albino rats. Unpublished report from Industrial Bio-Test Labs, Inc. to the Inter-Industry Color Committee, U.S.A. 1972. Summary in WHO/FAO 1975a, p. 13.

28. Holson, Jr., J.F., Gaylor, D.W., Schumaker, H.J., Collins, T.F.X., Ruggles, D.I., Keplinger, M.L., and Kennedy, Jr., G.L. Teratological Evaluation of FD and C Red. No. 2. A collaborative government-industry study. V. Combined findings and discussion. J. Toxicol. Environm. Hlth., 1: 875, 1976.

29. Holson, Jr., J.F., Schumaker, H.J., Gaylor, D.W., and Gaines, T.B. Teratological evaluation of FD and C Red No. 2. A colaborative government-industry study. IV. NCTR's study. J. Toxicol. Environm. Hlth., 1: 867, 1976.

30. Hooson, J., and Grasso, P. The effects of water-soluble chemicals on the growth of primary newborn rat kidney cells in culture. Toxicology, 7: 1-10, 1977.

31. Keplinger, M.L., Kinoshita, F.K., Smith, S.H., and Kennedy, Jr. G.L. Teratological evaluation of FD and C Red No. 2. A collaborative government-industry study. III. IBT's study. J. Toxicol. Environm. Hlth., 1: 863, 1976.

32. Keplinger, M.L., Wright, F.L., Plank, J.B., and Calandra, J.C. Teratologic studies with FD and C Red No. 2 in rats and rabbits. Toxicol. Appl. Pharmacol. 28: 209-215, 1974.

33. Khera, K.S., Przybylaski, W., and McKinley, W.P. Implantation and embryonic survival in rats treated with amaranth during gestation. Fd. Cosmet. Toxicol. 12: 507-510, 1974.

34. Khera, K.S., Roberts, G., Trivett, G., Terry, G. and Whalen, C. A teratogenicity study with amaranth in cats. Toxicol. Appl. Pharmacol. 38: 389-398, 1976.

35. Korinke, J., Taff, D., Smith, R.E., and Keplinger, M.L. Teratogenic and reproduction study with FD and C Red No. 2 in cats. Unpublished report from Industrial Bio-Test Labs. Inc. to Pet Food Institute, 1974. Summary in WHO/FAO 1975a, pp. 14-15.

36. Kugaczewska, M.M., and Krauze, S. Influence of some antioxidants, dyes, and artificial sweetening agents on metabolic processes of animal cells in vitro. Roczn. PZH. T. 23 (3): 165-171, 1972.

37. Larsson, K.S. A teratologic study with the dyes amaranth and ponceau 4R in mice. Toxicology, 4: 75-82, 1975.

38. Legator, M.S. Mutagenicity activity of FD and C Red No. 2 in the host-mediated assay. Unpublished report from the U.S. Food and Drug Administration, 1972. Summary in WHO/FAO 1975a, p. 15.

39. Lück, H., and Rickerl, E., Lebensmittelzusatzstoffe und mutagene Wirkung (Food additives and mutagenic effect). VI Report. Z. Leben-smitt.-Untersuch., 112: 157-174, 1960.

40. Manchon, Ph. and Albrecht, R. Comparison des effets du bordeaux S et du jaune de beurre chez le rat. Cah Notr. Diet., 7: 323-325, 1972.

41. Mannell, W.A., Grice, H.C., Lu, F.C., and Allmark, M.G. Chronic toxicity studies on food colours. IV. Observations on the toxicity of tartrazine, amaranth, and sunset yellow in rats. J. Pharm. Pharmacol. 10: 625- 34, 1958.

42. Mastalski, K., Jenkins, D.H., Plank, J.B., Kinoshita, F.K., Keplin-ger, M.L., and Calandra, J.C. Teratologic study in dogs, FD and C Red No. 2. Toxicol. Appl. Pharmacol. 33: 122, 1975.

43. Michaëlsson, G., and Juhlin, L. Urticaria induced by preservatives and dye additives in food and drugs. Brit. J. Dermatol. 88: 525-532, 1973.

44. Multigeneration study in the rat with amaranth. Unpublished report from the Food and Drug Administration, U.S.A., 1975. Summary in WHO/FAO 1975a, p. 19.

45. Nelson, A.A. and Hagan, E.C. Production of fibrosarcomas in rats at site of subcutaneous injection of various food dyes. Fed. Proc. 12: 397-398, 1953.

46. Newell, G.W., and Maxwell, W.A. Study of mutagenic effect of FD and C Red No. 2. Unpublished report (Compound report No. 1 and adden-dum) from the Stanford Research Institute submitted to the U.S. Food and Drug Administration, 1972. Summary in WHO/FAO 1975a, p. 15.

47. Parry, J.M. The use of yeast culture for the detection of environ-mental mutagens using a fluctuation test. Mut. Res., 46: 165-176, 1977.

48. Pritchard, A.B., Holmes, P.A., and Kirschman, J.C. The fate of FD and C Red No. 2 and its metabolite naphthionic acid after different routes of administration in the rat. Toxicol. Appl. Pharmacol. 35: 1-10, 1976.

49. Radomski, J.L., and Deichmann, W.B. Cathartic action and metabolism of certain coal-tar food dyes. J. Pharmacol. Exp. Ther., 118: 322-327, 1956.

50. Radomski, J.L., and Mellinger, T.J. The absorption, fate, and ex-cretion in rats of the water-soluble azo dye, FD and C. Red No. 2, FD and C Red No. 4 and FD and C Yellow No. 6. J. Pharmacol. Exp. Ther., 136: 259-266, 1962.

51. Reproduction and teratology studies in the hamster (amaranth). Un-published report from the Food and Drug Research Labs to the Food and Drug Administration, U.S.A., 1972. Summary in: WHO/FAO 1975a, p. 14.

52. Reproduction and teratology study in the mouse with amaranth. Un-published report from the Food and Drug Research Labs to the Food and Drug Administration, U.S.A., 1972. Summary in: WHO/FAO 1975a, p. 11.

53. Reproduction and teratology study in the rat with amaranth. Un-published report from the Food and Drug Research Labs to the Food and Drug Administration, U.S.A., 1972. Summary in: WHO/FAO 1975a, p. 13.

54. Roxon, J.J., Ryan, A.J., and Wright, S.E. Reduction of water-soluble azo dyes by intestinal bacteria. Fd. Cosmet. Toxicol. 5: 367-369, 1967.

55. Rubenchik, B.L. Enzyme activity in the liver of rats in carcinogene-sis induced by dimethylaminoazobenzene and following introduction of amaranth food colouring. Vop. Pitan., 21(5): 52, 1962. (Summary in Chem Abst., 58: 2717h).

56. Ryan, A.J., Roxon, J.J., and Sivayavirojana, A. Bacterial azo reduction: a metabolic reaction in mammals. Nature (London), 219: 854-855. 1968.

57. Ryan, A.J., and Wright, S.E. The excretion of some azo dyes in rat bile. J. Pharma. Pharmacol., 13: 492-495, 1961.

58. Sako, F., Taniguchi, N., Kobayashi, N., and Takakuwa, E. Effects of food dyes on Paramecium caudatum: toxicity and inhibitory effects on leucine aminopeptidase and acid phosphatase activity. Toxicol. Appl. Pharmacol., 39: 111-117, 1977.

59. Schumacher, H.J., Holson, J.F., Jr., and Gaines, T.B. Teratology study with FD and C Red No. 2. Unpublished report from the National Center for Toxicological Research, Jefferson, Arkansas, to the FDA ad hoc Advisory Group of the U.S. Food & Drug Administration, 1974. Summary in WHO/FAO 1975a, p. 12 (quoted as Anon., 1974a).

60. Seven-year toxicity study on female dogs with amaranth. Unpublished report from the Food and Drug Administration, U.S.A., 1974. Summary in: WHO/FAO 1975a, p. 19.

61. Shtenberg, A.I., and Gavrilenko, E.V. Influence of the food dye amaranth upon the reproductive function and development of progeny in test on albino rats. Vop. Pitan., 29(2): 66-73, 1970.

62. Shtenberg, A.I., and Gavrilenko, E.V. The gonadotoxic and embryotoxic effect of the food dye amaranth. Vop. Pitan., 31(5): 28-33, 1972.

63. Smith, S., Kennedy, G.L. Jr., and Keplinger, M.L. Teratology study with FD and C Red No. 2 in Charles River CD-1 albino rats. Unpublished report from Industrial Bio-Test Labs., Inc., submitted to the Inter-Industry Color Committee, U.S.A., 1974. Summary in WHO/FAO 1975a, p. 13.

64. Smith, S., Kennedy, G.L., Jr., and Keplinger, M.L. Fetal internal structural development. Teratology study with FD and C Red No. 2 in albino rats. Unpublished report from Industrial Bio-Test Labs., Inc., submitted to the Inter-Industry Color Committee, U.S.A., 1974. Summary in WHO/FAO 1975a, p. 13.

65. Sondergaard et al., 1977 (See allura red, Ref. 16).

66. Summary of toxicity studies on colours: amaranth (FD and C Red No. 2--Nos. 184 and 16185). Unpublished report from the Food and Drug Administration U.S.A. 1964. Summary in: WHO/FAO 1975a, pp. 17-18.

67. Truhaut, R., and Ferrando, R. Influence de l'administration, par voie orale, de différentes doses de deux colorants azoïques, l'amarante et le jaune soleil FCF, sur la mise en réserve de la vitamine A dans le foie du rat. C.R. Acad. Sci (Paris), 281(D,5): 459-462, 1975.

68. Willheim and Ivy, 1953 (See acid fuchsine, Ref. 4).

69. Winbush, J. Analysis of chick assay data on Red No. 2 and metabolites. Unpublished report (February, 8, 1972) to Dr. Verrett Submitted to WHO by the U.S. Food and Drug Administration, 1972. Summary in WHO/FAO 1975a, p. 16.

70. Holmberg, D. Effect of amaranth, ponceau 4R and/or vitamin A on enzyme activities of the rat liver. Fd. Cosmet. Toxicol. 16: 1-5, 1978.

ANNATTO

1. Durham, N.W., and Allard, R.K. A preliminary pharmacologic investigation of the roots of Bixa orellana. J. Amer. Pharm. Assoc. 49: 218-219, 1960.

2. Engelbreth-Holm, J., and Iverson, S. Is vegetable annatto butter colour carcinogenic? Acta Path. Microb. Scand., 37: 483-491, 1955.

3. Kay, J.H., and Calandra, J.C. One year chronic oral toxicity of aqueous annatto seed extract. Dogs. Unpublished report from Industrial Bio-Test Labs., Inc., submitted to the Marshall Dairy Lab., Inc., 1961. Summary in WHO/FAO 1975b, p. 44.

4. Lück and Rickerl, 1960 (See amaranth, Ref. 45).

5. Van Esch, G.J., van Genderen, H., and Vink, H.H. Über die chronische Verträglichkeit von Annatto farbstoff. Z. Lebensm.-Untersuch. 111: 93-108, 1959.

6. Zbinden, G., and Studer, A. Tierexperimentelle Untersuchungen über die chronische Verträglichkeit von beta-Carotin, Lycopin, 7,7'-Dihydro-beta-Carotin and Bixin. Z. Lebensm.-Untersuch., 108: 113-134, 1958.

ANTHOCYANINS

1. Alfieri, R., and Sole, P. Influence des anthocyanosides administrée par voie oro-perlinguale sur l'adopta-électroretinogramme (AERG) en lumière rouge chez l'homme. C.R. Soc. Biol., 160: 1590, 1966.

2. Horwitt, M.K. Observations on behavior of the anthocyan pigment from Concord grapes in the animal body. Proc. Soc. Exp. Biol. Med. 30: 949, 1933.

3. Jeney, E. Review and new data on the goitrogenic properties of flavonoids. Kiserl. Orvostud, 20: 514, 1968.

4. Kabiev, O.K., and Vermenichen, C.M. O protivoopukholevykh svoistvakh 3,5-diglikozid-tsianidina. Vopr. Onkol. 16: 80, 1970.

5. Lecomte, J., Sur les propriétés pharmacoligique des anthocyanosides du "Ribes nigrum" chez le rat. Thérapie, 29: 295-302, 1974.

6. Lietti, A., and Forni, G. Studies on Vaccinium myrtillus anthocyanosides. II. Aspects of anthocyanins pharmacokinetics in the rat. Arzneim.-Forsch, 26: 832-835, 1976.

7. Pourrat, H., Bastide, P., Dorier, P., Pourret, A., and Tronche, P. Preparation and therapeutic activity of some anthocyanin glycosides. Chem. Ther. 2: 33, 1967.

8. Sturua, A.Sh., Bokuchava, M.A., Baluiko, G.G., Erofeeva, N.N., and Siashvili, A.I. Biological action of the grape anthocyanin complex. Prokl. Biokhim. Mikrobiol. 7: 606-608, 1971.

9. Wegmann, R., Maeda, K., Tronche, P., and Bastide, P. Effects des anthocyanosides sur les photorécepteurs. Aspects cytoenzymologiques. Ann. Histochim. 14: 237-256, 1969.

AURAMINE

1. Acute toxicity in the mouse with auramine. Unpublished report from the Dept. of Pharmacology, Japanese National Institute of Hygienic Sciences, 1966.

2. Bonser, G.M. Precancerous changes in the urinary bladder. In: The Morphological Precursor of Cancer, Severi, L. (Ed.), Perugia, Italy, 1962.

3. Bonser, G.M., Clayson, D.B., and Jull, J.W. The induction of tumors of the subcutaneous tissues, liver and intestine in the mouse by certain dyestuffs and their intermediates. Brit. J. Cancer, 10: 653, 1956.

4. Case, R.A.M., and Pearson, J.T. Tumours of the urinary bladder in workmen engaged in the manufacture and use of certain dyestuff intermediates in the British chemical industry. Part II. Further con-

sideration of the role of aniline and of the manufacture of auramine and magenta (fuchsine) as possible causative agents. Brit. J. Industr. Med., 11: 213-216, 1954.

5. Green, H.N. Brit. Emp. Cancer Campaign, 39: 434, 1961.
6. Kawai, S. Toxicological study of coal-tar dyes. II. Their influence upon the isolated intestinal canal of rabbit and their relation to the chemical constitution. Kyoto J. Med. 25: 530-538, 1928.
7. Müller, A. von, Blasenveranderungen durch Amine, Erfahrungen aus dem Industriegebeit Basel. Z. Urol. Chir, 36:202, 1933.
8. Williams, M.H.C., and Bonser, G.M. Induction of hepatomas in rats and mice following the administration of auramine. Brit. J. Cancer, 16:87-91, 1962.
9. Walpole, A.L. On substances inducing cancer of the bladder. Acta Un. Int. Cancr., 19: 483, 1963.
10. Yao, M. Medical J. Osaka Univ., 36: 1485, 1937. Reported in J.L. Hartwell. Survey of compounds which have been tested for carcinogenic activity. Second Ed. 1951. National Cancer Institute, National Institute of Health. Bethesda, Md., p. 50.

AZORUBINE

1. Bär and Griepentrog, 1960 (see amaranth Ref. 14).
2. Bonser et al., 1956 (see auramine Ref. 3).
3. British Industrial Unpublished report (research report No. 8/1973) Biological Research Association, Carshalton, England, 1973. Summary in WHO/FAO 1975b, pp. 48-49.
4. DeMoor, H., Hendrickx, H., Casteels, M., Eekhout, W., and Buysse, F. Azorubine in commercial products and its presence in meat. Meded. Rijksfac. Landbouwwetensch, 34(4): 1067-1079, 1969.
5. Eisenbrand, J., and Pfeil, D., Über die Reduktion von Azofarbstoffen, insbesondere von Azorubin durch Milchsäurebäkterien. Naturwissenschaften, 42: 97-98, 1955.
6. Gaunt, I.F., Farmer, M., Grasso, P., and Gangolli, S.D. Acute (mouse and rat) and short-term (rat) toxicity studies on carmoisine. Fd. Cosmet. Toxicol., 5:179-185, 1967.
7. Gaunt, I.F., Grasso, P., Kiss, I.S., and Gangolli, S.D. Short-term toxicity study on carmoisine in the mini ture pig. Fd. Cosmet. Toxicol. 7: 1-7, 1969.
8. Goldblatt, and Frodsham, Unpublished report from Imperial Chemical Industries (ICI), England, 1952. Summary in WHO/FAO, 1975b, p. 48.
9. Hecht, G. Personal communication, Letter dated October, 13, 1966. Summary in WHO/FAO 1975b, p. 47.
10. Hecht, G., 1957 (see acid fuchsine FB, Ref. 1, p. 38).
11. Holmes, P., Pritchard, A.B., Kirschman, J.C. Multigeneration reproduction studies with carmoisine in rats. Toxicology, 10: 169-183, 1978.
12. Holmes, P.A., Pritchard, A.B., Kirschman, J.C. One year feeding study in rats. Toxicology, 10: 185-193, 1978.
13. Kugaczewska and Krause, 1972 (see Amaranth, Ref. 42).
14. Lück and Rickerl, 1960 (see amaranth, Ref. 45).
15. Mason, P.L., Gaunt, I.F., Butterworth, K.R., Hardy, J., Kiss, I.S., and Grasso, P. Long-term toxicity studies of carmoisine in mice. Fd. Cosmet. Toxicol., 12: 601-607, 1974.
16. Piekarski, L. Studies on affinity of dyes to protein from animal tissues. Part I. The method of the study. Roczn. PZH., 15: 283-293, 1964.

17. Ryan and Wright, 1961 (see amaranth, Ref. 59).

18. Sikorska and Krauze, 1962 (see acid fuchsine FB, Ref. 3).

19. Smith, J.M., Kasner, J.A. and Andresen, W. Carmoisine. Segment II. Rat teratology study. Unpublished report from Bio-Dynamics, Inc. submitted to the Inter-Industry Color Committee, U.S. 1972. Summary in WHO/FAO 1978 (to be issued).

20. Smith, J.M., Kasner, J.A. and Cannelongo, B., Segment II. Rabbit Teratology study. Unpublished report from Bio-Dynamics, Inc. Submitted to the Inter-Industry Color Committee, U.S.A., 1972. Summary in WHO/FAO 1978 (to be issued).

21. Vrbovsky, L., and Selecky, F.V. Pharmacological effects of dyes affecting the blood pressure. Bratislav Lekarske Listy, 39: 737-752, 1959.

22. Walker, R. The metabolism of azo compounds: a review of the literature. Fd. Cosmet. Toxicol. 8: 659-676, 1970.

BEET RED

1. Druckrey, H. Personal communication, 1959. Summary in WHO/FAO 1975, p. 51.

BENZYL VIOLET 4B

1. Gaunt, I.F., Hardy, J., Kiss, I.S., and Gangolli, S.D. Short-term toxicity of violet 6B (FD and C Violet No. 1) in the rat. Fd. Cosmet. Toxicol. 12: 11-19, 1974.

2. Grasso, P., Gangolli, S.D., Golberg, L., and Hooson, J. Physicochemical and other factors determining local sarcoma production by food additives. Fd. Cosmet. Toxicol., 9: 463-478, 1971.

3. Gangolli, S.D., Grasso, P., Golberg, L., and Hooson, J. Protein binding by food colourings in relation to the production of subcutaneous sarcoma. Fd. Cosmet. Toxicol. 10: 449-462, 1972.

4. Grasso, P., Hardy, J., Gaunt, I.F., Mason, P.L., and Lloyd, A.G. Long-term toxicity of violet 6B (Fd and C Violet No. 1) in mice. Fd. Cosmet. Toxicol., 12: 21-31, 1974.

5. Hess, S.M., and Fitzhugh, O.G. Metabolism of coal-tar colors. II. Bile studies (Abstract 1201). Fed. Proc., 13: 365, 1954.

6. Hess, S.M., and Fitzhugh, O.G. Absorption and excretion of certain triphenylmethane colors in rats and dogs. J. Pharmacol Exp. Ther., 114:38-42, 1955.

7. Ikeda, Y., Horiuchi, S., Imoto, A., Kodama, Y., Aida, Y., and Kobayashi, K. Induction of mammary gland and skin tumour in female rats by the feeding of benzyl violet 4B. Toxicology, 2: 275-284, 1974.

8. Lu, F.C. and Lavallée, A. The acute toxicity of some synthetic colours used in drugs and foods. Canad. Pharm. J., 97: 30, 1964.

9. Mannell, W.A., Grice, H.C., and Allmark, M.G. Chronic toxicity studies on food colours. V. Observations on the toxicity of brilliant blue FCF, guinea green B, and banzyl violet 4B in rats. J. Pharm. Pharmac., 14: 378-384, 1962.

10. Mannell, W.A., Grice, H.C., and Dupuis, I. The effect on rats of long-term exposure to guinea green B and benzyl violet 4B. Fd. Cosmet. Toxicol. 2: 345-347, 1964.

11. Minegishi, K.I., and Yamaha, T. Metabolism of triphenylmethane colours. II. Absorption, excretion and distribution of benzyl violet 4B (FD and C Violet No. 1) in rats. Toxicology, 7: 367-383, 1977.

12. Nelson, A.A., and Davidow, B. Injection site fibrosarcoma production in rats by food colors (Abstract No. 1571). Fed. Proc., 16: 367, 1957.
13. Radomski and Deichmann, 1956 (see amaranth, Ref. 54).
14. Tullar, P.E., Unpublished report from George Washington University, 1947. Summary in WHO/FAO 1978 (to be issued).
15. Uematsu, K., and Miyaji, T. Induction of tumours in rats by oral administration of technical acid violet 6B. J. Nat. Canc. Inst. 51: 1337-1338.

BLACK 7984

1. Hecht, G. Personal communication, 1960. Summary in WHO/FAO 1978 (to be issued).
2. Hecht, G. Quoted in R. Truhaut. Estratto dei Rendiconti dell'Istituto Superiore di Sanita', 25: 796-920, 1960.
3. Hecht, G., and Wingler, A. Biological study and suitable chemical constitution of some azo dyes for food colourings. Arzneimittel.-Forsch. 2: 192-196, 1952.
4. Gangolli et al., 1972 (see benzyl violet 4B, Ref. 4).
5. Sondergaard et al., 1977 (see allura red, Ref. 16).

BLUE VRS

1. Clayson, D.B., Pringle, J.A.S., Bonser, G.M., and Wood, M. The technique of bladder implantation: further results and an assessment. Brit. J. Cancer, 22: 825-832, 1968.
2. Dacre, J.C. Synthetic organic food colours: toxicology and biochemical aspects. Fd. Technology. N.Z., 4: 169-177, 1969.
3. Farbwerke Hoechst, A.G. Unpublished Report October 1964.
4. Grasso et al., 1971 (see benzyl violet 4B, Ref. 3).
5. Gangolli et al., 1972 (see benzyl violet 4B, Ref. 4).
6. Gangolli, S.D., Grasso, P., and Golberg, L. Physical factors determining the early local tissue reactions produced by food colourings and other compounds injected subcutaneously. Fd. Cosmet. Toxicol. 5:601-621, 1967.
7. Grasso, P., and Golberg, L. Early changes at the site of repeated subcutaneous injection of food colourings. Fd. Cosmet. Toxicol. 4: 269-282, 1966.
8. Grice, H.C., and Mannell, W.A. Rhabdomyosarcom s induced in rats by intramuscular injections of blue VRS. J. Nat. Cancer Inst. 37: 845-857, 1966.
9. Grice, H.C., Dupuis, I., Dennery, M., and Mannell, W.A. Blue VRS-induced rhabdomyosarcomas (Abstract No. 25). Toxicol. Appl. Pharmacol., 8: 342-343, 1966.
10. Hall, D.E., Gaunt, I.F., Farmer, M., and Grasso, P. Acute (mouse and rat) and short-term (rat) toxicity studies on blue VRS. Fd. Cosmet. Toxicol. 5: 165-170, 1967.
11. Hooson, J., Grasso, P., and Gangolli, S.D. Injection site tumours and preceeding pathological changes in rats treated subcutaneously with surfactants and carcinogens. Brit. J. Cancer, 27: 230-244, 1973.
12. Mannell, W.A., and Grice, H.C., Chronic toxicity of brilliant blue FCF, blue VRS, and green S in rats. J. Pharma. Pharmacol. 16: 56-59, 1964.

13. Miller, E.W., Brit. Emp. Cancer Campaign, 34: 312, 1956.
14. Miller, E.W., and Pybus, F.C. Brit. Emp. Cancer Campaign, 32: 246, 1954.
15. Williams, M.H.C. Communication delivered to a Symposium in Tokyo, typewritten document dated December 1964.

BRILLIANT BLACK PN

1. Bär and Griepentrog, 1960 (see amaranth, Ref. 14).
2. Diemair, W., and Boeckhoff, K. Brilliant Black BN: Künstliche Farbstoffe und Fermentreaktionen. 4. Ihr Einfluss auf Trypsin und Duodenalsaft. Z. Analyt. Chem., 139: 35-37, 1953.
3. Diemair, W., and Hausser, H. Synthetic dyes and enzyme reaction. Z. Lebensm.-Untersuch. u.-Forsch. 92: 165-170, 1951.
4. Drake, J.J-P., Butterworth, K.R., Gaunt, I.F., and Grasso, P. Long-term toxicity study of black PN in mice. Fd. Cosmet. Toxicol. 15: 503-508, 1977.
5. Gaunt, I.F., Carpanini, F.M.B., Grasso, P., and Kiss, I.S. Long-term feeding study on black PN in rats. Fd. Cosmet. Toxicol. 10: 17-27, 1972.
6. Gaunt, I.F., Colley, J., Creasey, M., and Grasso, P. Short-term toxicity of black PN in pigs. Fd. Cosmet. Toxicol., 7: 557-567, 1969.
7. Gaunt, I.F., Farmer, M., Grasso, P., and Gangolli, S.D. Acute (mouse and rat) and short-term (rat) toxicity studies on black PN. Fd. Cosmet. Toxicol. 5: 171-177, 1967.
8. Hecht, 1957 (see Acid fuchsine FB, Ref. 1, p. 58).
9. Hecht, G., and Wingler, A. Die biologische Untersuchung und der geeignete chemische Aufbau einiger Azofarbstoffe zur Lebensmittelfärbung. Arzneimittel.-Forsch. 2: 192-196, 1952.
10. Kugaczewska and Krauze, 1972 (see amaranth, Ref. 42).
11. Lang, E. Cleavage products of the azo dyes, brilliant black BN, yellow orange S, orange GGN, and their effect on acid production by lactic acid bacteria. Z. Lebensm.-Unters. Forsch., 132: 363-367, 1967.
12. Lück and Rickerl, 1960 (see amaranth, Ref. 45).
13. Piekarski, L. Studies on the absorption of brilliant black BN from the alimentary canal of the rat. Roczn. Zak. Hig. (Warsz), 11: 353-356, 1960.
14. Ryan, A.J., and Welling, P.G. The metabolism and excretion of black PN in the rat and man. Fd. Cosmet. Toxicol., 8:487-497, 1970.
15. Saenz, L.R., and Laroche, C. Note sur la reduction du noir brillant BN chauffé en presence du sucres et sur la formation des colorants monoazoiques qui en derivant. Ann. Fals. Exp. Chim., 53: 581, 1960.
16. Sikorska and Krauz, 1962 (see acid fuchsine FB, Ref. 3).

BRILLIANT BLUE FCF

1. Brilliant blue FCF: additional information. Unpublished report from Imperial Chemical Industries (ICI), England 1962. Summary in WHO/FAO 1970, p. 25.
2. Daniel, J.W. The excretion of some triphenylmethane food colours by the rat: brilliant blue FCF. Unpublished report from Imperial Chemical Industries (ICI), England, 1958. Summary in WHO/FAO 1970, p. 24.

3. Despopoulos, 1968 (see amaranth, Ref. 25).
4. Gangolli et al. 1972 (see benzyl violet 4B, Ref. 4).
5. Graham and Allmark, 1959 (see amaranth, Ref. 32).
6. Grasso and Golberg, 1966 (see blue VRS, Ref. 7).
7. Gross, E. Production of sarcomas with purified triphenylmethane dyes light green SF and patent blue AE upon repeated subcutaneous injection into rats. Z. Krebsforsch., 64: 287-304, 1961.
8. Hansen, W.H., Fitzhugh, O.G., Nelson, A.A., and Davis, K.J. Chronic toxicity of two food colors, brilliant blue FCF and indigotine. Toxicol. Appl. Pharmacol., 8:29-36, 1966.
9. Hess, S.M., and Fitzhugh, O.G. Brilliant blue FCF—Metabolism of coal-tar dyes. I. Triphenylmethane dyes. Fed. Proc., 12: 330-331, 1953.
10. Hess and Fitzhugh, 1954 (see benzyl violet 4B, Ref. 6).
11. Hess and Fitzhugh, 1955 (see benzyl violet 4B, Ref. 7).
12. Iga, T., Awazu, S., and Nogami, H. Pharmacokinetic study of biliary excretion. II. Comparison of excretion behavior in triphenylmethane dyes. Chem. Pharm. Bull., 19: 273-281, 1971.
13. Iga, T., Awazu, S., Hanano, M., and Nogami, H. Pharmacokinetic studies of biliary excretion. IV. The relationship between the biliary excretion behavior and the elimination from plasma of azo dyes and triphenylmethane dyes in rats. Chem. Pharm. Bull., 19: 2609-2616, 1971.
14. Klinke, J. Unpublished results quoted in Ref. 1 (see acid fuchsine FB, Ref. 1, p. 73).
15. Lu and Lavallée, 1964 (see benzyl violet 4B, Ref. 9).
16. Mannell and Grice, 1964 (see blue VRS, Ref. 12).
17. Mannell et al., 1962 (see benzyl violet 4B, Ref. 10).
18. Nelson and Hagan, 1953 (see amaranth, Ref. 50).
19. Rowland, I.R., Gaunt, I.F., Hardy, J., Kiss, I.S., and Butterworth, K.R. Long-term toxicity of brilliant blue FCF in mice. Fd. Cosmet. Toxicol. (In press).
20. Sako et al., 1977 (see amaranth, Ref. 60).
21. Summary of toxicity studies on colours: brilliant blue FCF (FD and C Blue No. 1). Unpublished report from the U.S. Food and Drug Administration, 1969. Summary in WHO/FAO 1970, p. 24.
22. Willheim and Ivy, 1953 (see acid fuchsine FB, Ref. 4).

BROWN FK

1. An investigation of the acute and sub-acute toxicity of brown FK with associated pathological and metabolic studies. Unpublished report from the British Industrial Biological Research Association (BIBRA) (Research report No. 5/1964), 1964. Summary in WHO/FAO 1978a (to be issued).
2. Ashmole, R.T., Campbell, P., Kirkby, W.W., and Wilson, R. Effects of feeding dietary brown FK to rats for 6 and 16 weeks. Unpublished report from Unilever Ltd. 1966. Summary in WHO/FAO 1978a (to be issued).
3. Ashmole, R.T., Kirkby, W.W., and Wilson, R. Thirteen-week mouse feeding trial. Unpublished report from Unilever Ltd., 1958. Summary in WHO/FAO 1978a (to be issued).
4. Edwards, K.B., and Wilson, R. Acute toxicity of brown FK in rats, mice, guinea pigs, rabbits, and chickens. Unpublished report from unilever Ltd. 1966. Summary in WHO/FAO 1978a (to be issued).
5. Fore, H., and Walker, R. Studies of brown FK. I. Composition and synthesis of components. Fd. Cosmet. Toxicol., 5: 1-9, 1967.

6. Fore, H., Walker, R., and Golberg, L. Studies on brown FK. II. Degradative changes undergone in vitro and in vivo. Fd. Cosmet. Toxicol., 5: 459-473, 1967.
7. Fuller, A.T. Is p-aminobenzenesulphonamide the active agent in prontosil therapy? Lancet, Jan. 23, pp. 194-198, 1937.
8. Gaunt, I.F., Hall, D.E.,Grasso, P., and Golberg, L., Studies on brown FK. V. Short-term feeding studies in the rat and pig. Fd. Cosmet. Toxicol. 6:301-312, 1968.
9. Goldblatt and Frodsham, 1952 (see azorubine, Ref. 8).
10. Grasso, P., and Golberg, L. Problems confronted and lessons learned in the safety evaluation of brown FK. Fd. Cosmet. Toxicol. 6, 737-747, 1968.
11. Grasso, P., Gaunt, I.F., Hall, D.E., Golberg, L., and Batstone, E. Studies on brown FK. III. Administration of high doses to rats and mice. Fd. Cosmet. Toxicol. 6: 1-11, 1968.
12. Grasso, P., Muir, A., Golberg, L., and Batstone, E. Studies on brown FK. IV. Cytopathic effects of brown FK on cardiac and skeletal muscle in the rat. Fd. Cosmet. Toxicol., 6: 13-24, 1968.
13. Hope, J. Ultrastructure of the pigment induced in various tissues of the rat by long-term feeding of the dye brown FK. Unpublished rep rt from Unilever Ltd., 1971. Summary in WHO/FAO 1978a (to be issued).
14. Howes, D. Metabolism of ^{14}C labelled i,3-diamino-4-(p-sulphophenylazo)benzene, a component of the dye brown FK, in the rat. Unpublished report from Unilever Ltd., 1969. Summary in WHO/FAO 1978a (to be issued).
15. Kirkby, W.W. Nature of the pigment induced in tissues of rats and mice fed brown FK. Unpublished report from Unilever Ltd., 1968. Summary in WHO/FAO 1978 (to be issued).
16. Kirkby, W.W. Effects of brown FK and two of its constituents on pigment deposition and lesions in rats and mice. Unpublished report from Unilever Ltd., 1968. Summary in WHO/FAO 1978a (to be issued).
17. Jenkins, F.P., and Favell, D.J. Metabolism of the monoazobenzene component of brown FK in human subjects. Unpublished report from Unilever Ltd., 1971. Summary in WHO/FAO 1978a (to be issued).
18. Müller, E., Über ein Oxydationsprodukt des Tri-amidobenzols. Chem. Ber. 22: 856, 1889.
19. Munday, R. Metabolism of 2,4-diamino-5-(p-sulphophenylazo) toluene. Unpublished report from Unilever Ltd., 1969. Summary in WHO/FAO 1978a (to be issued).
20. Mulky, M.J., Munday, R., Ashmole, R.T., and Kirkby, W.W. Evaluation of the terminal causative agent in Brown FK induced myopathy and pigment deposition. Unpublished report from Unilever Ltd., 1969. Summary in WHO/FAO 1978a (to be issued).
21. Munday, R. Uncoupling of oxidative phosphorylation by Brown FK metabolites. Unpublished report from Unilever Ltd., 1971. Summary in WHO/FAO 1978a (to be issued).
22. Munday, R., and Kirkby, W.W. Metabolism of 1,3-diamino-4-(p-sulphophenylazo)benzene. Unpublished report from Unilever Ltd., 1969. Summary in WHO/FAO 1978a (to be issued).
23. Venitt, S., and Bushell, C.T. Mutagenicity of the food colour Brown FK and constituents in S. typhimurium. Mutation Res. 40: 309-316, 1976.
24. Walker, R., Grasso, P., and Gaunt, I.F. Myotoxicity of amine metabolites from Brown FK. Fd. Cosmet. Toxicol. 8: 539-542, 1970.
25. Wilson, R., Gellatly, J.B.M., Kirkby. W.W., and Ashmole, R.T., Biological evaluation of Brown FK: 80-week mouse feeding trial. Un-

published report from Unilever Ltd., 1970. Summary in 1978a (to be issued).

26. Wilson, R., Gellatly, J.B.M., Kirkby, W.W., and Ashmole, R.T. Biological evaluation of Brown FK: 2-year rat feeding trial. Unpublished report from Unilever Ltd., 1971. Summary in WHO/FAO 1978a (to be issued).

BUTTER YELLOW

1 Hartwell, J.L. Survey of compounds which have been tested for carcinogenic activity. Washington D.C. U.S. Government Printing Office (Public Health Service Publication No. 149), 1951.

2. Shubik, P., and Hartwell, J.L. Survey of compounds which have been tested for carcinogenic activity. Washington D.C., U.S. Government Printing Office (Public Health Service Publication No. 149; Supplement 1) 1957.

3. Shubik, P. and Hartwell, J.L. Survey of compounds which have been tested for carcinogenic activity. Washington D.C. U.S. Government Printing Office (Public Health Service Publication N. 149: Supplement 2), 1969.

CANTHAXANTHINE

1. Essais de toxicité avec la canthaxanthine. Unpublished report from Hoffman La Roche. Summary in WHO/FAO 1975b, p. 57.

CARAMEL

1. A short-term (10-week) feeding study with three caramels in rats. Unpublished report from BIBRA (report No. 177/2/77), 1977. Summary in WHO/FAO 1978a (to be issued).

2. A study of the haematological effects of caramel in human volunteers. Unpublished report from the British Industrial Biological Research Association (report No. 1/172/76), 1976. Summary in WHO/FAO 1978a (to be issued).

3. Bachmann, G., Haldi, J., Wynn, W., and Ensor, C. Reproductivity and growth of albino rats on a prolonged daily intake of caffeine. J. Nutr. 32: 307-320, 1946.

4. Bartlett, S., and Broster, W.H. Feeding trials with ammoniated molasses in the diet of young dairy cattle. J. Agric. Sci., 50: 60-63, 1958.

5. Brusick, D. Mutagenic evaluation of compound FDA 71-83 (caramel). Unpublished report from Litton Bionetics, Inc. (project Dec. LBI/2468), 1974. Summary in WHO/FAO 1978a (to be issued).

6. Chacharonis, P. Acute and chronic toxicity study on caramel colours A and B. Unpublished report from Scientific Associated, Inc. to the Union Starch and Refining Co. Columbus, Indiana, 1960. Summary in WHO/FAO 1975b, p. 60.

7. Chacharonis, P. Acute and subacute oral toxicity study in rats on caramel colourings 25A-1,30B-0, and 30F-1. Unpublished report from Scientific Associates, Inc. to the Union Starch and Refining Co., Granite City, Ill. 1963, Summary in WHO/FAO 1975b, p. 60.

8. Chronic (2- year) toxicity study with rats. Unpublished report from TNO. The Netherlands, submitted to WHO by the Ad hoc Technical Caramel Committee 1972. Summary in WHO/FAO 1975b, p. 60.

9. Evans, J.G., Butterworth, K.R., Gaunt, I.F., and Grasso, P. Longterm toxicity study in the rat on a caramel produced by the half

open/half closed pan ammonia process. Fd. Cosmet. Toxicol. 15:523-531, 1977.

10. Foote, W.L., Robeinson, R.F., and Davidson, R.S. Toxicity of caramel color products (102 B, 103 B, 104 B, 107 B, 108 B, 109 B, and 110 B). Unpublished report from Battelle Memorial Institute, Colombus, Ohio, to the Union Starch and Refining Co., Inc., 1968. Summary in WHO/FAO 1975b, p. 60.

11. Fuji, S., Tsuchida, H., and Komoto, M. Chemical studies on the reaction products of glucose and ammonia. Part X. Isolation and Identification of 4(5)-(DL-glycero-2,3-dihydroxypropyl)imidazole. Agric. Biol. Chem. 30: 73-77, 1966.

12. Gaunt, I.F., Lloyd, A.G., Grasso, P., Gangolli, S.D., and Butterworth, K.R. Toxicological investigations of caramel I.A. short-term study in the rat with two caramels produced by variations of the ammonia process. Unpublished report from BIBRA, (report No. 14/1975), 1975. Summary in WHO/FAO 1978a (to be issued).

13. Gaunt, I.F., Lloyd, A.G., Grasso, P., Gangolli, S.D., and Butterworth, K.R. Short-term study in the rat on two caramels produced by variations of the ammonia process. Fd. Cosmet. Toxicol. 15: 509-521, 1977.

14. Haldi, J., Wynn, W., and Shelfon, W.H. A study to determine whether or not caramel has any harmful physiological effect. Unpublished report from Emory University, Atlanta, Ga., to the Coca-Cola Co., Atlanta, Ga., 1951, Summary in: WHO/FAO 1975b, p. 61.

15. Haldi, J., Wynn, W., and Sheldon, W.H. A study to determine whether or not caramel has any harmful physiological effect. Experiment 73-X. Unpublished report from Emory University, Atlanta, Ga. The Coca-Cola Co., Atlanta, Ga., 1958. Summary in WHO/FAO 1975b, p. 61.

16. Heyns, K., Unpublished report from the Ad Hoc Techincal Caramel Committee, 1970. Summary in WHO/FAO 1975b, p. 59.

17. Heyns, K. Unpublished report from the Ad Hoc Technical Caramel 1971. Summary in WHO/FAO 1975a, p. 59.

18. Hough, L., Jones, J.K.N., and Richards, E.L. The reaction of amino-compounds with sugars. The reaction of ammonia and d-glucose. J. Chem. Soc., pp. 3854-3857, 1952.

19. Kay, J.H., and Calandra, J.C. Subacute oral toxicity of caramel colourings in dogs and rats. Unpublished report from Inudstrial Bio-Test Labs, Inc., Northbrook, Ill., to the Corn Products Refining Co., Argo, Ill., US, 1962. Summary in WHO/FAO 1972a, pp. 61-62.

20. Komoto, M. Chemical research on the reaction products of glucose and ammonia. I. Changes occurring in glucose in aqueous ammonia solution. J. Agric. Chem. Soc. Japan, 36: 305-310, 1962.

21. Loeper, M., Mougeot, A., and Parrod, J. L'action hydropigène de quelques imidazols. C.R. Soc. Biol. 118: 405-406, 1935.

22. Marier, G., and Orr, J.M. Tolerance study of double strength sulfite caramel in human volunteers. Unpublished report (report No. 5711) from Bio-Research Labs., 1977. Summary in WHO/FAC 1978a (to be issued).

23. Marier, G., and Orr, J.M. Tolerance study of single strength ammonia sulfite caramel in human volunteers. Unpublished report (project No. 5612) from Bio-Research Labs, Canada, 1977. Summary in WHO/FAO 1978a (to be issued).

24. Morgareidge, K. Teratologic evaluation of FDA 71-83 (caramel, beverage) in mice, rats, and rabbits. Unpublished report from the Food and Drug Research Labs., Inc. (report No. PB 234-867), 1974. Summary in WHO/FAO 1978a (to be issued).

25. Morgareidge, K. Teratologic evaluation of FDA 71-82 (caramel, bakers, and confectioners) in mice, rats, and rabbits. Unpublished report from the Food and Drug Research Lab., Inc. (report No. PB 234-870.), 1974. Summary in WHO/FAO 1978a (to be issued).

26. Nees, P.O. Toxicological feeding study of caramel E. Unpublished report from the Wisconsin Alumni Research Foundation, Madison, Wis., Submitted to the Pepsi-Cola Co., Long Island City, N.Y., 1964. Summary in WHO/FAO 1975b, p. 62.

27. Nishie, K., Waiss Jr., A.C., and Keyl, A.C. Toxicity of methyli-midazoles. Toxicol. Appl. Pharmacol. 14: 301-307, 1969.

28. Nishie, K., Waiss, Jr. A.C., and Keyl, A.C. Pharmacology of alkyl and hydroxyalkylpyrazines. Toxicol. Appl. Pharmacol. 17: 244-249, 1970.

29. Oser, B.L. Toxicological feeding study of acid-proof caramel. Unpublished report from the Food and Drug Research Labs., Inc., N.Y., submitted to the Williamson and Co., Inc., Long Island City, N.Y., 1963. Summary in WHO/FAO 1975b, p. 62.

30. Prier, R.F. The toxicity of double strength acid proof caramel in rats—12-week feeding test. Unpublished report from the Wisconsin Alumni Research Foundation, Madison, Wis., submitted to the Sethness Products Co., Keokuk, Iowa, 1960. Summary in WHO/FAO 1975b, p. 61.

31. Procter, B.G. A preliminary evaluation of the potential toxico-logical effects of ammonia caramel in mice. Unpublished report from Bio-Research Labs., Ltd. Canada (project no. 5705), 1979. Summary in WHO/FAO 1978a (to be issued).

32. Procter, B.G., Berry, G., and Chappel, C.I. A toxicological evalua-tion of various caramels fed to albino rats. Unpublished report (project No. 4244) from Bio-research Labs., Canada, 1976. Summary in WHO/FAO 1978a (to be issued).

33. Sharratt, M. British Industrial Biological Research Association (BIBRA) safety evaluation program: caramels. Private communica-tion from the author, 1971. Summary in WHO/FAO 1975b, pp. 60 and 62.

34. Sinkeldam, E.J., and Van der Heyden, C.A. Short-term feeding study with caramel SS 202 in albino rats. Unpublished report (report No. R4777) from CIVO-TNO, The Netherlands, 1975. Summary in WHO/FAO 1978a, (to be issued).

35. Sinkeldam, E.J., and Van der Heyden, C.A. Short-term feeding test with three types of caramels in albino rats. Unpublished report (report No. R4789) from CIVO-TNO, The Netherlands, 1975. Summary in WHO/FAO 1978a (to be issued).

36. Sinkeldam, E.J., and Van der Heyden, C.A. Short-term (10-week) feeding study in rats with three different ammonia caramels. Un-published report (report No. R5120) from CIVO-TNO, The Netherlands, 1976. Summary in WHO/FAO 1978a (to be issued).

37. Sinkeldom, E.J., Van der Heyden, C.A., and Beems, R.B. Chronic (2-year) feeding study in rats with six different ammonia caramels. Unpublished report (report No. R4961) from CIVO-TNO, The Netherlands, 1976. Summary in WHO/FAO 1978a (to be issued).

38. Sinkeldam, E.J. Willems, M.I., and Van der Heyden, C.A. One-year feeding study in rats with six different ammonia caramels. Unpub-lished report (report No. R4767) from CIVO-TNO, The Netherlands, 1975. Summary in Who FAO 1978a, (to be issued).

39. Til, H.P., and Spanjers, M.Th., Reproduction study in rats with six different ammonia caramels. Unpublished report from CIVO-TNO (report No. R4068), The Netherlands, 1973. Summary in WHO/FAO 1978a (to be issued).

40. Wiggins, L.F. Some recent studies on ammoniated molasses. Sugar, J., 18: 18-20, 1956.
41. Warner, J.S. Topical report on determination of 4-methylimidazole in caramel color samples. Unpublished report from Battelle Memorial Institute, Columbus, Ohio, submitted to the Ad hoc Technical Caramel Committee of Industrial Manufactuers and Users. Summary in WHO/ FAO 1975b, p. 59 (quoted as Batelle).

CARBON BLACKS

1. Almquist, H.J., and Zandler, D. Absorbing charcoald in chick diets. Proc. Soc. Exp. Biol. Med., 45: 303-306, 1940.
2. Capusan, I., and Mauksch, J. Cutaneous affections associated with the manufacture of carbon black. Berufsdermatosen. 17(1): 28 37, 1969.
3. Disselbeck, F. There are no carcinogenic hazards regarded in manufacturing carbon black since 1930. Internal statement of the author to Degussa, 1976.
4. Falk, H., Kotin, L., and Mehler, P. Polycyclic hydrocarbons as carcinogens for man. Arch. Environm. Hlth. 8: 721, 1964.
5. Gabor, S., Raucher, C., Stefanescu, A., Ossian, A., and Corne , G.H. Occupational hazards in the carbon black industry. Igiena, 18(1): 57-62, 1969 (Chem. Abstr. 71, 63844, 1969).
6. Ingalls, T.H. Incidence of cancer in the carbon black industry, Arch. Ind. Hyg. and Occ. Med. 26(1): 662, 1950.
7. Ingalls, T.H., and Resquez-Iribarren, R. Periodic search for cancer in the carbon black industry. Arch. Environm. Hlth., 2: 429, 1961.
8. MacCallum, D.K., Patek, P.R., and Bernick, S. Pulmonary arterial reactions to experimentally produced carbon emboli. Arch. Path. 81: 509-513, 1966.
9. Metzger, K.B., Soot toxicology. A small "white book" for carbon black. Chem.-Ztg. 100(1): 15-24, 1976.
10. Nau, C.A., Neal, J., and Stembridge, V. A study of the physiological effects of carbon black ingestion. A.M.A. Arch. Ind. Hlth. 17: 21-28, 1958.
11. Neal, J., Stembridge, V., and Nau, C.A. A study of the physiological effects of carbon black. Arch. Industr. Hlth. 18: 511, 1958.
12. Nau, C.A., Neal, J., and Stembridge, V.A. A study of the physiological effects of carbon black. Arch. Environm. Hlth., 1: 512, 1960.
13. Nau, C.A., Neal, J., Stembridge, V.A., and Cooley, R.N. Physiological effects of carbon black. Arch. Environm. Hlth. 4: 415, 1962.
14. Radomski, J.L. Unpublished report to the American Toilet Goods Association, 1968.
15. Rigdon, R.H. Tissue reaction to foreign materials. CRC Crit. Rev. Tox. 3(4): 435-476, 1975.
16. Steiner, P.E. The conditional biological activity of the carcinogens in carbon blacks, and their elimination. Cancer Res. 14: 103, 1954.
17. Tara, S. Carbon Black. Rev. Path. Gen. Phys. Clin. (France), 718: 643-775, 1960.
18. Tomingas, R. Untersuchung über die Schädlichkeit von Russen unter besonderer Berückchtigung ihrer cancerogenen Wirkung, 4. Mitteilung: Russimplantation und Sarkome bei Ratten. Staub.-Reinh. Luft. 27: 347, 1967.

19. Tsuchiya, K. The relation of occupation to cancer, especially cancer of the lung. Cancer, 18: 136-144, 1965.
20. Udagawa, T. Response of albino rat lung to a carcinogenic hydrocarbon. Experimental induction of pulmonary tumours. (Japanese text), Ochanomizu Med. J., 7: 2103, 1959 (Excerpta Med. Amst. 9: 5459, 1961.
21. Von Haam, E., and Allette, F.S. Studies on the Toxicity and Skin effects of compounds used in the rubber and plastics industries. III. Carcinogenicity of carbon black extracts. AMA Arch. Ind. Hyg. Occup. Med., 6: 237, 1952.
22. Von Haam, E., Titus, H.L., Caplan, I. and Shinowara, G.Y. Effect of carbon blacks on carcinogenic compounds. J. Occ. Med. 1:418, 1959.
23. Valic, F., Beritic-Stahuljak, D. and Mark, B. A follow-up study of functional and radiological lung changes in carbon black exposure. Int. Arch. Arbeitsmed., 34(1): 51-63, 1975.

BETA-APO-8'-CAROTENAL

1. Bagdon, R.E., Impellizzeri, C., and Osadca, M. Studies on the toxicity and metabolism of beta-apo-8'-carotenal in dogs. Toxicol. Appl. Pharmacol., 4: 444-456, 1962.
2. Bagdon, R.E., Zbinden, G., and Studer, A. Chronic toxicity studies of beta-carotene. Toxicol. Appl. Pharmacol., 2: 225-236, 1960.
3. Beta-apo-8'-carotenal. Unpublished report from Hoffmann La Roche, 1962. Summary in WHO/FAO 1975b, p. 66.
4. Brubacher, G., Gloor, U., and Wiss, O. Zum Stoffwechsel von beta-apo-8'-carotenal (C_{30}), Chimia, 14, 19-20, 1960.
5. Glover, J. The conversion of beta-carotene into vitamin A. Vit. Horm., 18: 371-385, 1960.
6. Thommen, H. Recherches sur le metabolisme de l'apo-8'-caroténal. Chimia, 15, 433-434, 1961.
7. Tiews, J. Vitamin A-Wirksamkeit der Carotine bei verschiedenen Tierarten. Dtsch. Gesellsch. Ernährung., 9: 235-262, 1963.
8. Travaux originaux cités dans la documentation sur les caractéristiques physico-chimiques, le dosage, l'emploi et les propriétes biologiques du beta-apo-8'-caroténal. Unpublished report from Hoffmann La Roche, 1966. Summary in WHO/FAO 1975b, p. 66.
9. Wiss, O., and Thommen, H. Stoffwechsel der Carotine. Dtsch. Gesellsch. Ernährung., 9: 179-192, 1963.
10. Wood, J.D. The hypocholesterolemic activity of beta-apo-8'-carotenal. Canad. J. Biochem., 41: 1663-1665, 1963.

BETA-CAROTENE (NATURAL AND SYNTHETIC)

1. Abrahamson, I.A., Sr., and Abrahamson, I.A., Jr. Hypercarotenemia. Arch. Ophth., 66: 34-37, 1962.
2. Auckland, G. A case of carotenaemia. Brit. Med. J., 2: 267-268, 1952.
3. Bagdon et al., 1960 (see beta-apo-8'-carotenal, ref. 4).
4. Bernhard, K. Resorption von Carotinen und Carotinoiden. Wiss. Veroff. Dtsch. Gesellsch. Ernährung, 9: 169-177, 1963.
5. Beta-carotene. Unpublished report from Hoffmann La Roche, 1960. Summary in WHO/FAO 1975b, p. 69.
6. Brubacher et al., 1960 (see beta-apo-8'-carotenal, ref. 5).
7. Brubacher, G., Schärer, K., Studer, A., and Wiss, O. Über die gegenseitige Neeninflussung von Vitamin E, Vitamin A, und Carotinoiden. Z. Ernährung, 5: 190-202, 1965.

8. Fraps, G.S. and Meinke, W.W. Digestibility by rats of alpha and beta and neo-beta-carotenes in vegetables. Arch. Biochem., 6: 323-327.
9. Greenberg, R., Cornbleet, T., and Joffay, A.I. Accumulation and excretion of vitamin-A-like fluorescent material by sebaceous glands after the oral feeding of various carotenoids. J. Invest. Dermat., 32: 599-604, 1959.
10. Kübler, W., Carotine in der säuglingsernahrung. Wiss. Veröff. Gesellsch. Ernährung., 9: 222-234, 1963.
11. Nieman, C., and Klein-Obbink, H.J. The biochemistry and pathology of hypervitaminosis A. Vit. Horm., 12: 69-99, 1954.
12. Wagner, K. Zum Problem des Karotinpseudoikterus. Wien. Klin. Wschr. 74: 909-213, 1962.
13. Zbinden and Studer, 1958 (see annatto, Ref. 6).

BETA-APO-8'-CAROTENOIC ACID

1. Essais de toxicité avec les esters méthylique et éthylique de l'acide beta-apo-8'-caroténoïque. Unpublished report from Hoffmann La Roche, 1964. Summary in WHO/FAO 1975b, p. 72.
2. Kübler, 1963 (see beta-carotene, Ref. 10).
3. Travaux originaux cités dans la documentation sur les caractéristiques. Physico-chimiques, le dosage, l'emploi et les propriétes biologiques du beta-apo-8'-caroténal. Unpublished report from Hoffmann La Roche, 1966. Summary in WHO/FAO 1975b, pp. 72-73.
4. Wiss and Thommen, 1963 (see beta-apo-8'-carotenal, Ref. 9).

CARTHAMUS

1. Chiba, S. Subacute toxicity of yellow dye Tanacolor-y [R] (carthamus yellow). Unpublished report from Juntendo University School of Medicine, Dept. of Public Health, Tokyo, Japan, submitted to Tanabe Seiyaku Co., Ltd., Osaka, Japan, 1970. Summary in WHO/FAO 1978a, (to be issued).
2. Chiba, S. Chronic toxicity of Tanacolor-y [R](carthamus yellow). Unpublished report from Juntendo University School of Medicine, Dept. of Public Health, Tokyo, Japan, submitted to Tanabe Seiyaku Co., Ltd., Osaka, Japan, 1972. Summary in WHO/FAO 1978a (to be issued).
3. Kuwamura, Ikeda, and Ishihara, Acute toxicity of carthamus yellow. Unpublished report from the research staff of Tanabe Seiyaku submitted to Tanabe Seiyaku., Ltd., Osaka, Japan, 1970. Summary in WHO/FAO 1978a (to be issued).

CHLOROPHYLLS, CHLOROPHYLLINS, AND COPPER COMPLEXES

1. Brugsch, J.T. and Sheard, C. Determination and quantitative estimation of decomposition of chlorophyll in human body. J. Lab. Clin. Med., 24: 230-240, 1938.
2. Campbell, I.R., Cass, J.S., Chlak, J., and Kehoe, R.A. Aluminum in the environment of man. Arch. Med. Assoc. Ind. Hlth., 15: 359-448, 1957.
3. Harrison, J.W.E., Levin, S.E., and Trabin, B. The safety and fate of potassium sodium copper chlorophyllin and other copper compounds. J. Amer. Pharm. Assoc. Sc. Ed., 43: 722-737, 1954.
4. Heinrichs, D., Rummel, W., and Schunk, R. Zur Pharmakologie des Chlorophylls. Arzneimittel.-Forsch., 4: 19-20, 1954.

5. Levshin, B.J. Farmakologiceskaja harakteristika preparatove hloro-
   fillina natrii. Farmakol. i Toksikol. 21: 46-51, 1958.
6. Reber, E.F., and Willigan, D.A. The effects of a chlorophyll derivative when included in a ration fed rats. II. reproduction,
   blood, and tissue studies. Amer. J. Vet. Res., 15: 643-646, 1954.
7. Tomino, U. Experimental histopathological studies on the biological
   action of sodium-copper chlorophyllin (in Japanese). Kobe Ika Daig-
   aku Kiyo, 14: 98-119, 1958.
8. Worden, A.N., Bunyan, J., and Kleissner, M., Toxicity studies on
   sodium copper chlorophyllin. Brit. Vet. J., 111: 385-387, 1955.

CHOCOLATE BROWN FB

1. Butterworth, K.R., Gaunt, I.F., Grasso, P., and Gangolli, S.D.
   Short-term toxicity of chocolate brown FB in pigs. Unpublished report from BIBRA (report No. 3/1975), 1975. Summary in WHO/FAO
   1978a, (to be issued).
2. Fore et al., 1967 (see Brown FK, Ref. 6).
3. Gaunt, I.F., Brantom, P.G., Grasso, P., and Kiss, I.S. Long-term
   studies of chocolate brown FB in mice. Fd. Cosmet. Toxicol. 11:
   375-382, 1973.
4. Gaunt, I.F., Brantom, P.G., Grasso, P., Creasey, M., and Gangolli,
   S.D. Long-term feeding study on chocolate brown FB in rats. Fd.
   Cosmet. Toxicol. 10: 3-15, 1972.
5. Gaunt, I.F., Hall, D.E., Farmer, M., and Fairweather, F.A. Acute
   (mouse and rat) and short-term (rat) toxicity studies on chocolate
   brown FB. Fd. Cosmet. Toxicol., 5: 159-164, 1967.
6. Goldblatt and Frodsham, 1952 (see azorubine, Ref. 8).

CHOCOLATE BROWN HT

1. Carpanini, F.M.B., Butterworth, K.R., Gaunt, I.F. Kiss, I.S., Grasso,
   P., and Gangolli, S.D. Long-term toxicity studies on chocolate
   brown HT in rats. Unpublished report from the BIBRA (report 19/
   1975), 1975. Summary in WHO/FAO 1978a (to be issued).
2. Chambers, P.L., Hunter, C.G., and Stevenson, D.E. Short-term study
   of chocolate brown HT in rats. Fd. Cosmet. Toxicol., 4: 151-155,
   1966.
3. Drake, J.J-P., Butterworth, K.R., Gaunt, I.F., and Hardy, J. Long-
   term toxicity studies of chocolate brown HT in mice. Unpublished
   report from the BIBRA (Research report No. 16/1975), 1975. Summary
   in WHO/FAO 1978a (to be issued).
4. Fore et al. 1967 (see Brown FK, Ref. 6).
5. Hendy, R.J., Butterworth, K.R., Gaunt, I.F., Hooson, J., and Grasso,
   P. Short-term toxicity study of chocolate brown HT in pigs. Unpublished report from the BIBRA (research report No. 17/1975), 1975.
   Summary in WHO/FAO 1978a, (to be issued).
6. Walker, R., 1970 (see azorubine, Ref. 22).
7. Hall, D.E., Lee, F.S., and Fairweather, F.A. Acute (mouse and rat)
   and short-term (rat) toxicity studies on chocolate brown HT. Fd.
   Cosmet. Toxicol., 4: 143-149, 1966.

CHRYSOIDINE

1. Albert, Z. Induction of adenomas and carcinomas in the liver of mice
   by prolonged feeding with chrysoidine (in Polish). Excerpta Med.
   (Amst.) Sect.16(3): 2177, 1955.
2. Albert, Z. Effect of prolonged feeding with chrysoidin on the formation of adenomas and cancer of the liver in mice. Arch. Immunol.
   Ter. Dosw., 4: 189-242, 1956.

3. Cambel, P., Breindenbach, A.W., and Ray, F.E. A physio-pathological study of the rat's stomach and blood after administration of chrysoidine Y and alpha-azurine. Amer. J. Physiol. 178: 493-498, 1954.
4. Kinosita, R. Researches on carcinogenesis of various chemicals (in Japanese). Gann, 30: 423-426, 1936.
5. Kinosita, R. Studies on carcinogenic azo and related compounds. Yale J. Biol. Med., 12: 287-300, 1940.
6. Krauze, S., Piekarski, L., and Suslow, A. Studies on affinity of dyes to animal proteins. Rocz. Panstw. Zakl. Hig., 15: 1-3, 1964.
7. Kugaczewska and Krauze, 1972 (see amaranth, Ref. 42).
8. Maruya, M. On the renal changes of albino rats induced by the oral administration of 14 azo-compounds and 5 aromatic amino-compounds. Tr. Jap. Path. Soc., 28: 541-547, 1938.
9. Nitti, F., and Bovet, D. Recherches expérimentelles sur les phénomènes allergiques provoqués par la sulfamidochrysoidine. Rev. Immunol., 2: 460-464, 1936.
10. Piekarski, L., and Marciszewski, H. Affinity of carcinogenic chrysoidine for proteins of mice liver. Rcz. Panstw. Zakl. Hig., 17: 485-489, 1966.
11. Sikorska and Krauze, 1962 (see acid fuchsine FB, Ref. 3).

CHRYSOINE S

1. Bär and Griepentrog, 1960 (see amaranth, Ref. 14).
2. Hech, 1955 (see acid fuchsine FB, Ref. 1, p. 26).
3. Luck and Rickerl, 1960 (see amaranth, Ref. 45).
4. Sondergaard and Hansen, 1977 (see allura red, Ref. 16).
5. Waterman, N. and Lignac, G.O.E. Long-term study in mice. Summary in Acta Physiol. Pharmacol. Neerl., 7: 35, 1958.
6. Zsolnai, T. Versuch zur Entdeckung neuer Fungistatika. VI. Hydrazin-Derivate und organische Basen bzw, ihre Salze. Biochem. Pharmacol., 11: 995-1016, 1962.

CHRYSOINE SGX "SPECIALLY PURE"

1. Druckrey, H., Schädliche und unsschädliche Farbstoffe fur Lebensmittel. Z. Krebsforsch., 60:344-360, 1955.
2. Druckrey, H., and Hamperl, H., Klin. Wschr. 28: 289, 1950.
3. Hecht, G., 1955, (see acid fuchsine FB, Ref. 1, p. 31).
4. Klinke, 1955 (see brilliant blue FCF, Ref. 15).

CITRANAXANTHIN

1. Hempel, K.J. Results of macroscopical and microscopical investigations in chronic toxicity tests on rats with citranaxanthin. Unpublished report.
2. Kawase, S., Komatsu, Y., Suzuki, Y., Nishida, S., Kobayshi, A., Subacute toxicity of citranaxanthin. J. Med. Soc. Toho., (Japan), 19: 499-504, 1972.
3. Kolk, J.H.H. About vitamin A efficiency and pigmenting effect of three citranaxanthin preparations in chicks and quails with different crystal size. Dissertation, University Munich, FRG, 1974.
4. Leuschner, F. Investigation of acute toxicity of citranaxanthin with dogs, 1976. Unpublished report.
5. Leuschner, F., Leuschner, A., Schwerdtfeger, W., and Dontenwill, W. Investigation of chronic toxicity (2-year) of citranaxanthin with rats, 1976. Unpublished report.

6. Leuschner, F., Leuschner, A., Schwerdtfeger, W., and Dontenwill, W., 6-month toxicity of citranaxanthin with beagle dogs by administration in feed, 1975. Unpublished report.
7. Leuschner, F., Hubscher, F., and Dontenwill, W. Investigation of chronic toxicity of citranaxanthin in a 3-generation study with rats, 1976. Unpublished report.
8. Tiews, J. Certified report about vitamin A activity of citranaxanthin and other carotenoids, Munich, 1978. Unpublished report.
9. Zeller, H. Results of acute toxicity investigations, 1972. Unpublished report.
10. Zeller, H., Kirsch, P., Koop, K., and Freisberg, K.O. Report on the examination of citranaxanthin dry powder, 10 percent, in a 91-day feeding test with rats, 1973. Unpublished report.

CITRUS RED 2

1. Clayson et al. 1968 (see blue VRS, Ref. 2).
2. Dacre, J.C. Chronic toxicity and carcinogenicity studies on citrus red No. 2. Proc. Univ. Otago Med. Sch., 43: 31-33, 1965.
3. Paynter, O.E., and Scala, R.A. Chronic and subcutaneous toxicity of (2,5-dimethoxyphenylazo)-2-naphthol (citrus red 2). Unpublished report from Hazleton Labs., Falls Church, Va., 1964. Summary in WHO/FAO 1970, pp. 30-31.
4. Radomski, J.L. The absorption, fate, and excretion of citrus red No. 2 (2,5-dimethoxyphenyl-azo-2-naphthol) and Ext. D and C Red No. 14 (1-xylylazo-2-naphthol). J. Pharmacol. Exp. Ther., 134: 100-109, 1961.
5. Radomski, J.L., 1-amino-2-naphthyl glucoronide, a metabolite of 2,5-dimethoxy-2-naphthol and 1-xylylazo-2-naphthol. J. Pharmacol. Exp. Ther., 136: 378-385, 1962.
6. Sharratt, M. Frazer, A.C., and Paranjoti, I.S. Biological effects of citrus red No. 2 in the mouse. Fd. Cosmet. Toxicol., 4: 493-502, 1966.

COCHINEAL/CARMINE/CARMINIC ACID

1. Brown, J.P., and Brown, R.J. Mutagenesis by 9.10-anthraquinone derivatives and related compounds in S. Typhimurium. Mutat. Res., 40: 203-224, 1976.
2. Brown, J.P., Roehm, G.W., and Brown, R.J. Mutagenicity testing of certified food colours and related azo, xanthene and triphenylmethane dyes with Salmonella/microsome system. 8th Annual Meeting Environmental Mutagen Society, Colorado Springs, February, 1977 (abstract).
3. Gaunt, I.F., Clode, S.A., and Lloyd, A.G. Studies of the teratogenicity and embryotoxicity of carmine in the rat. Unpublished report from the BIBRA, 1976. Summary in WHO/FAO 1978a (to be issued).
4. Harada, M. cited by Hartwell, J.L.: Survey of Compounds Which Have Been Tested for Carcinogenicity Activity. Second Edition, 1951, p. 118, 1931.
5. Kada, T., Tutikawa, K., and Sadaie, Y. In vitro and host-mediated rec-assay procedures for screening chemical mutagens; and phloxine, a mutagenic red dye detected. Mut. Res., 16: 165-174, 1972.
6. Luck and Rickerl, 1960 (see amaranth, Ref. 45).
7. Oser, B.L. A 90-day feeding study with carmine. Unpublished report from the Food and Drug Research Labs, to H. Kobnstamm and Co., Inc., New York., 1962. Summary in WHO/FAO 1975b, p. 78.
8. Sarkany, R.H., Meara, R.H., and Everall, J. Cheilitis due to carmine in lip salve. Trans. St. John's Hosp. Derm. Soc., 48: 30-40, 1961.

9. Schlüter, G. Über die embryotoxische Wirkung von Carmin bei der Maus (Embryotoxic action of carmine in mice). Z. Anat. Entwickl.-Gesch., 131: 228-235, 1970.
10. Schlüter, G. Time-response relationship of embryotoxic effects of lithium carmine in mice. Naunyn-Schmiedebergs Arch. Pharmak. 270: 316-318, 1971.
11. Schlüter, G. Effects of lithium carmine and lithium carbonate on the prenatal development of mice (in German). Naunyn-Schmiedebergs Arch. Pharmak., 270:56-64, 1971.
12. Surber, W. Subacute toxicity study of cochineal red in rats. Unpublished report from Battelle Memorial Institute, Geneva, Switzerland submitted to D. Campari, S.p.a., Milan, Italy. Summary in WHO/FAO, 1975b, p. 78.

CONGO RED

1. Beaudoin, A.R. Teratogenicity of congo red in rats. Proc. Soc. Exp. Biol., 117: 176-179, 1964
2. Bedaux, F.C., Bruining, M., and Meijers, C.A.M., Pharm. Weekbl., 97: 213, 1962.
3. Richardson, A.P., and Dillon, J.K., Jr. Congo red: toxicity and systemic action. Amer. J. Med. Sci., 198: 73-82, 1939.
4. Somers, G.F., and Whittet, T.D. British Pharmaceutical Conference Dublin, p. 21, 1956.
5. Taliaferro, I., and Haag, H.B. Toxicity and effect of congo red upon blood coagulation. Amer. J. Med. Sci., 193: 626-633, 1937.
6. Weyl, T. The Coal Tar Colours (German Edition). Berlin, 1889.

EOSINE

1. Calnan, C.D., Z. Haut.-u.Geschl.-Kr., 27: 61, 1959.
2. Daels, F.C.R. Congress on Cancer, Strasbourg, 1923. Summary in Ref. 1 (acid fuchsine FB, p. 90).
3. Gangolli et al., 1972 (see benzyl violet 4B, Ref. 4).
4. Hansen, W.H., Fitzhugh, O.G., and Williams, M.W. Subacute oral toxicity of nine D and C coal-tar colors (Abstract No. 7789), J. Pharmacol. Exp. Ther., 122: 29A, 1958.
5. Hecht, G. 1957 (see acid fuchsine FB, Ref. 1, (p. 90).
6. Hellier, F.F., Lipstick dermatitis: with report of case due to eosin. Brit. J. Derm., 49: 485-491, 1937.
7. Hiller, F.K. Prüfung des tetrabromfluoresceins (Eosinsäure) auf Verträglichkeit und Cancerogenität. Arzneimittel-Forsch., 12: 587-588, 1962.
8. Iga, T., Awazu, S., and Nogami, H. Pharmacokinetic study of biliary excretion. III. Comparison of excretion behavior in xanthene dyes, fluorescein, and bromsulphthalein. Chem. Pharm. Bull., 19: 297-308, 1971.
9. Kada, T., Mutagenicity testing of chemicals in microbial systems. In: Coulston, F. et al., eds. New Methods in Environmental Chemistry and Toxicology, Tokyo, Academic Scientific Books, pp. 127-133, 1973.
10. Kugaczewska and Krauze, 1972 (see amaranth, Ref. 42).
11. Lück, H., Wallnofer, P., and Bach, H., Lebenmittelzusatzstoffe und mutagene Wirkung. VII. Mitteilung. Prüfung einiger Xanthen-Farbstoffe auf mutagene Wirkung an E. coli. Path. et Microbiol. (Basel), 26: 206-224, 1963.
12. NIOSH (National Institute for Occupational Safety and Health), 1976. Registry of Toxic Effects of Chemical Substances, Rockville, Md. U.S. Department of Health, Education and Welfare, p. 542.
13. Sako et al., 1977 (see amaranth, Ref. 60).

14. Sikorska and Krauze, 1962 (see acid fuchsine FB, Ref. 3).
15. Umeda, M., Rat sarcoma produced by the injection of eosine yello-wish. Gann. 46: 367-368, 1955.
16. Umeda, M., Experimental study of xanthese dyes as carcinogenic agents. Gann, 47: 51-78, 1956.
17. U.S. Food and Drug Administration, 1964. Summary in WHO/FAO, 1978 (to be issued).
18. Webb, J.M., Fonda, M., and Brouwer, E.A. Metabolism and excretion patterns of fluorescein and certain halogenated fluorescein dyes in rats. J. Pharmacol. Exp. Ther., 137: 141-147, 1962.
19. Willheim and Ivy, 1953 (see acid fuchsine FB, Ref. 4).

ERYTHROSINE

1. Andersen, C.J., Keiding, N.R., and Nielson, A.B. False elevation of serum protein-bound-iodine caused by red colored drugs or foods. Scand. J. Clin. Lab. Inrest., 16: 249, 1964.
2. Bär and Griepentrog, 1960 (see amaranth, Ref. 14).
3. Bowie, W.C., Wallace, W.C., and Lindstrom, H.V. Some clinical mani-festations of erythrosine in rats. Fed. Proc., 25: 556 (Abstract 2079), 1966.
4. Butterworth, K.R., Gaunt, I.F., Grasso, P., and Gangolli, S.D. Acute and short-term toxicity studies on erythrosine BS in rodents. Fd. Cosmet. Toxicol., 14: 525-531, 1976.
5. Butterworth, K.R., Gaunt, I.F., Grasso, P., and Gangolli, S.D. Short-term toxicity of erythrosine BS in pigs. Fd. Cosmet. Toxicol., 14: 533-536, 1976.
6. Collins, T.F.X., and Long, E.L. Effects of chronic oral administra-tion of erythrosine in the mongolian gerbil. Fd. Cosmet. Toxicol., 14: 233-248, 1976.
7. Daniel, J.W. The excretion and metabolism of edible food colors. Toxicol. Appl. Pharmacol., 4: 572-594.
8. Dickinson, D. and Raven, T.W. Stability of erythrosine in artificial-ly coloured canned cherries. J. Sci. Food Agric., 13: 650-652, 1962.
9. Diemair and Hausser, 1951 (see brilliant black BN, Ref. 3).
10. Emerson, G.A., and Anderson, H.H. Toxicity of certain proposed anti-leprosy dyes: fluorescein, eosin, erythrosin, and others. Int. J. Leprosy, 2: 257-263, 1934.
11. Graham, and Allmark, 1959 (see amaranth, Ref. 32).
12. Grasso and Golberg, 1966 (see blue VRS, Ref. 7).
13. Haley, S., Three-generation reproduction study with FD and C Red No. 3 in albino rats. Unpublished report from Industrial Bio-Test Labs, Inc., Northbrook, Ill., submitted to the Inter-industry Color Committee 1972. Summary in WHO/FAO 1975b, p. 81.
14. Haley, S., Kennedy, G.L., Jr. and Keplinger, M.L. Rabbit teratology study. Unpublished report from Industrial Bio-Test Labs, Inc. North-brook, Ill., submitted to the Inter-Industry Color Committee 1973. Summary in WHO/FAO 1975b, p. 82.
15. Haley, S., Kennedy, G.L., Jr., and Keplinger, M.L. Three-generation reproduction study with FD and C Red No. 3 (erythrosine) in albino rats. Unpublished report from Industrial Bio-Test Labs, Inc., North-brook, Ill., submitted to the Inter-Industry Color Committee. Sum-mary in WHO/FAO 1975b, p. 82.
16. Hansen, W.H., Davis, K.J., Graham, S.L., Perry, C.H., and Jacobson, K.H. Long-term toxicity studies of erythrosine. II. Effects on haematology and thyrosine and protein-bound iodine in rats. Fd. Cos-met. Toxicol., 11: 535-545, 1973.

17. Hansen, W.H., Zwickey, R.E., Brouwer, J.B., and Fitzhugh, O.G. Long-term studies of erythrosine. I. Effects in rats and dogs. Fd. Cosmet. Toxicol., 11: 527-534, 1973.
18. Hung, W. Elevation of protein-bound iodine in an 8-year old due to transplacental passage of an organic iodine dye. Pediatrics, 37: 677-680, 1966.
19. Kugaczewska and Krauze, 1972 (see amaranth, Ref. 42).
20. Lu and Lavallée, 1964 (see benzyl violet 4B, Ref. 9).
21. Lück and Rickerl, 1960 (see amaranth, Ref. 45).
22. Lück et al., 1963 (see eosine, Ref. 13).
23. Marignan, R., Boucard, M., and Gelis, C. Influence possible de l'érythrosine sur le metabolisme thyroidien. Trav. Soc. Pharm. (Montpellier), 24: 127-130, 1965.
24. Nelson and Hagan, 1953 (see amaranth, Ref. 50).
25. Payne, J.V. Benign red pigmentation of stool resulting from food coloring in a new breakfast cereal (the Franken Berry Stool), Pediatrics, 49: 293-294, 1972.
26. Sako et al., 1977 (see amaranth, Ref. 60).
27. Sikorska and Krauze, 1962 (see acid fuchsine FB, Ref. 3).
28. Tanaka, K., and Ckahara, K. Effects of food additives on the alimentary tract. J. Food Hyg. Soc., 14: 234-238, 1973.
29. Umeda, 1956 (see eosine, Ref. 17).
30. Vought, R.L., Brown, F.A., and Wolff, J. Erythrosine: an adventitious source of iodine. J. Clin. Endocr. Met., 34: 747-752, 1972.
31. Waliszewski, T. Chromatographic and biological investigation of food stuff colouring matters (in Polish). Acta Pol. Pharm., 9: 127-148, 1952.
32. Waterman and Lignac, 1958 (see chrysoine, Ref. 5).
33. Webb et al., 1962 (see eosine, Ref. 18).
34. Willheim and Ivy, 1953 (see acid fuchsine FB, Ref. 4).

FAST GREEN FCF

1. Gangolli et al., 1967 (see blue VRS, Ref. 6).
2. Gangolli et al., 1972 (see benzyl violet 4B, Ref. 4).
3. Grasso and Golberg, 1966 (see blue VRS, Ref. 7).
4. Hansen, W.H., Long, E.L., Davis, K.J., Nelson, A.A., and Fitzhugh, O.G. Chronic toxicity of three food colorings: guinea green B, light green SF yellowish, and fast green FCF in rats, dogs and mice. Fd. Cosmet. Toxicol., 4: 389-410, 1966.
5. Hess and Fitzhugh, 1953 (see brilliant blue FCF, Ref. 10).
6. Hess and Fitzhugh, 1955 (see benzyl violet 4B, Ref. 7).
7. Hess and Fitzhugh, 1954 (see benzyl violet 4B, Ref. 6).
8. Hesselbach, M.L., and O'Gara, R.W. Fast green- and light green-induced tumours: induction, morphology , and effect on host. J. Nat. Cancer Inst., 24: 769-793, 1960.
9. Iga et al., 1971 (see brilliant blue FCF, Ref. 13).
10. Lu and Lavallée, 1964 (see benzyl violet 4B, Ref. 9).
11. Nelson and Hagan, 1953 (see amaranth, Ref. 50).
12. Radomski and Deichmann, 1956 (see amaranth, Ref. 54).
13. Sako et al., 1977 (see amaranth, Ref. 60).
14. Willheim and Ivy, 1953 (see acid fuchsine FB, Ref. 4).

FAST RED E

1. Bär and Griepentrog, 1960 (see amaranth, Ref. 14).
2. Diemair and Hausser, 1951 (see brilliant black BN, Ref. 3).

3. Gross, E. Unpublished results. Summary in Ref. 1 (acid fuchsine) p. 39.
4. Hecht, G. Unpublished results. Summary in Ref. 1 (acid fuchsine) p. 39.
5. Lück and Rickerl, 1960 (see amaranth, Ref. 45).
6. Specifications for fast red E. Fd. Cosmet. Toxicol., 6: 370-371, 1968.
7. Waterman and Lignac, 1958 (see chrysoine, Ref. 5).

FAST YELLOW AB

1. Bar and Griepentrog, 1960 (see amaranth, Ref. 14).
2. Diemair and Hausser, 1951 (see brilliant black BN, Ref. 3).
3. Evstatieva, M. Toxicological evaluation of new dyes during a subacute study in animals. Khig Zdraneopaz., 17(3): 287-291, 1974.
4. Gross, E. Unpublished results. Summary in Ref. 1 (acid fuchsine) p. 23.
5. Hecht, G. Unpublished results. Summary in Ref. 1 (acid fuchsine) p. 23.
6. Hromatka, O., Stentzel, L., and Broda, E., Über die Synthese von radioaktiv markiertem Echtgelb (1'-14C'4'aminoazobenzol-3-4'-disulfonsaürem Natrium). Monatshefte fur Chemie, 86 (3): 444, 1955.
7. Karrer, K., Broda, E., Stark, R., Hromatka, O., and Zischka, W. Metabolism experiments with radioactive disodium 4-aminoazo-benzene-3,4'-disulfonate. (see Ref. 6).
8. Klinke, J. Unpublished results. Summary in Ref. 1 (acid fuchsine) p. 23.
9. Kugaczewska and Krauze, 1972. (see amaranth, Ref. 42).
10. Luck and Rickerl, 1960 (see amaranth, Ref. 45).
11. Ryan and Wright, 1961 (see amaranth, Ref. 59).
12. Scheline, R.R., and Longberg, B. The absorption, metabolism and excretion of the sulphonated azo dye acid yellow by rats. Acta Pharmaco. Tox. 23: 1-14, 1965.
13. Scheline, R.R., Nygaard, R.T., and Longberg, B. Enzymatic reduction of the azo dye, acid yellow, by extracts of Streptococcus faecalis isolated from rat intestine. Fd. Cosmet. Toxicol., 8: 55-58, 1970.
14. Sikorska and Krauze, 1962 (see acid fuchsine, Ref. 3).
15. Sondergaard et al., 1977 (see allura red, Ref. 16).

FERROUS GLUCONATE

1. Carr, C.J. Evaluation of the health aspects of iron and iron salts as food ingredients. Life Science Research Office. Federation of American Societies for Experimental Biology, Bethesda, Md., 1973.
2. Carr, C.J.,, Patrick J., Jr., and Waddell, J. The bioavailability of iron sources and their utilization in food inrichment. Life Science Research Office. Federation of American Societies for Experimental Biology, Bethesda, Md., 1973.
3. Hoppe, J.O., Agnew-Marcelli, G.M., and Tainter, M.L. An experimental study of the toxicity of ferous gluconate. Am. J. Med. Sci., 230: 491-498, 1955.
4. Iron and Iron salts used in foods. Summary of bibliographical data from Informatics, Inc. Rockville, Md. 1973.
5. Pfizer Ltd, 1967. Summary in WHO/FAO 1975a, p. 26. Unpublished report.

FOOD GREEN S

1. Dalgaard-Mikkelsen, S.V., and Rasmussen, F. Tracer dyes for rapid detection of antibiotics in milk. 16th International Dairy Congress, pp. 465-473, 1962.
2. Daniel, J.W. Unpublished report submitted by Imperial Chemical Industries, 1959. Summary in WHO/FAO 1975b, p. 89.
3. Lu and Lavallée, 1964 (see benzyl violet 4B, Ref. 9).
4. Mannell and Grice, 1964 (see blue VRS, Ref. 12).
5. Toxicity studies with green S in the rat and the mouse. Unpublished report from Imperial Chemical Industries, 1964. Summary in WHO/FAO 1975b, p. 90.
6. Truhaut, R. Unpublished report from the author, 1964. Summary in WHO/FAO 1975b, pp. 91-92.

GOLD

1. Block, W.D., Buchanan, O.H., and Freyberg, R.H. A comparative study of the distribution and excretion of gold following intramuscular injection of five different gold compounds. J. Pharmac. Exp. Ther. 23: 200-204, 1941.
2. Freyberg, R.H., Block, W.D., and Levey, S., Human plasma and synovial fluid concentration and urinary excretion of gold during and following treatment with gold sodium thiomalate and gold sodium thiosulfate and colloidal gold sulphate. J. Clin. Invest., 20: 401-412, 1941.
3. Kleinsorge, H., Corvens, H.J., Dornbusch, S., and Dresslee, E. Untersuchungen uber Resorption, Ablagerung und Auscheidung von Goldsalzen im Organismus unter Verwendung von radioactive Gold (198 Au). Allergie, Asthma, 5:217-224, 1959.
4. Krusius, F.E., Markkanen, A., and Peltola, P. Plasma levels and urinary excretion of gold during routine treatment of rheumatoid arthritis. Ann. Rheum. Dis., 29: 232-235, 1970.
5. Petering, H.G. Pharmacology and toxicology of heavy metals: gold. Pharmac. Ther., 1: 119-125, 1976.
6. Stube, J. and Galle, P. Role of mitochondria in the handling of gold by the kidney. J. Cell. Biol., 44: 667-676, 1969.
7. Thompson, H.E. Gold toxicity in rheumatoid arthritis. Ariz. Med. 31 (12): 912-915, 1974.

GUINEA GREEN B

1. Graham and Allmark, 1959 (see amaranth, Ref. 32).
2. Hansen et al., 1966. (see fast green FCF, Ref. 4).
3. Hess and Fitzhugh, 1953 (see brilliant blue FCF, Ref. 10).
4. Hess and Fitzhugh, 1954 (see benzyl violet 4B, Ref. 6).
5. Hess and Fitzhugh, 1955 (see benzyl violet 4B, Ref. 7).
6. Iga et al., 1971 (see brilliant blue FCF, Ref. 13).
7. Lu and Lavallée, 1964 (see benzyl violet, Ref. 9).
8. Mannell et al., 1962 (see benzyl violet 4B, Ref. 10).
9. Mannell et al., 1964 (see benzyl violet 4B, Ref. 11).
10. Minegishi, K.I., and Yamaha, T. Metabolism of triphenylmethane colors. I. Absorption, excretion, and distribution of guinea green B (FD and C Green No. 1) in rats. Chem. Pharm. Bull., 22: 2042-2047, 1974.
11. Nelson and Hagan, 1953 (see amaranth, Ref. 50).
12. Willheim and Ivy, 1953 (see acid fuchsine FB, Ref. 4).

INDANTHRENE BLUE RS

1. Bar and Griepentrog, 1960 (see amaranth, Ref. 14).
2. Klinke, J. Unpublished results. Summary in Ref. 1 (acid fuchsine, p. 104).
3. Lu and Lavellée, 1964 (see benzyl violet 4B, Ref. 9).
4. Nothdurft, H. Unpublished results. Summary in Ref. 1 (acid fuchsine P. 104).
5. Oettel, H., Frohberg, H., Nothdurft, H., and Wilhelm, G. Die Prüfung einiger synthetischer Farbstoffe auf ihre Eignung zur Lebensmittelfärbung. Arch. Toxikol., 21: 9-29, 1965.
6. Umeda, 1956 (see eosine, Ref. 17).

INDIGOTINE

1. Bär and Griepentrog, 1960 (see amaranth, Ref. 14).
2. Gaunt, I.F., Kiss, I.S., Grasso, P., and Gangolli, S.D. Short-term toxicity study on indigo carmine in the pig. Fd. Cosmet. Toxicol. 7: 17-24, 1969.
3. Graham and Allmark, 1959 (see amaranth, Ref. 32).
4. Hansen et al., 1966 (see billiant blue FCF, Ref. 9).
5. Hooson, J., Gaunt, I.F., Kiss, I.S., Grasso, P., and Butterworth, K.R. Long-term toxicity of indigo carmine in mice. Fd. Cosmet. Toxicol. 13: 67-176, 1975.
6. Kempton, R.R., Bott, P.A., and Richards, A.N. The glomerular elimination of indigo carmine in rabbits. Amer. J. Anat., 61: 505-518, 1937.
7. Kugaczewska and Krauze, 1972 (see amaranth, Ref. 42).
8. Lethco, E.J. and Webb, J.M. The fate of FD and C Blue No. 2 in rats. J. Pharmacol. Exp. Ther., 154: 384-389, 1966.
9. Lu and Lavallée, 1964 (see benzyl violet 4B, Ref. 9).
10. Lück and Rickerl, 1960 (see amaranth, Ref. 45).
11. Oettel et al., 1965 (see indanthrene blue RS, Ref. 5).
12. Sikorska and Krauze, 1962 (see acid fuchsine, Ref. 3).
13. Summary of toxicity studies: indigotine. Unpublished report from the U.S. Food and Drug Administration, 1969. Summary in WHO/FAO 1975b, p. 96.
14. Wazeter, F.X., Goldenthal, E.I., Geil, R.G., and Harris, S.D. Multigeneration reproduction study in rats. Unpublished report from the International Research and Development Corporation to the Inter-Industry Color Committee, 1974. Summary in WHO/FAO 1975b, p. 96.
15. Wazeter, F.X., Goldenthal, E.I., Geil, R.G., and Harris, S.B. Rabbit teratology study. Unpublished report from the International Research and Development Corporation, Mattawan, Mich., to the Interindustry Color Committee 1972. Summary in WHO/FAO 1975b, p. 96.

IRON OXIDES AND HYDRATED IRON OXIDES

1. IARC monographs on the evaluation of carcinogenic risk of chemicals to man. International Agency for Research on Cancer, Vol. 1, 29-39, 1972.
2. Iron metabolism, Lancet (1): 428-429, 1963.
3. Steinhoff, D., Personal communication, 1972. Summary in WHO/FAO 1975b, p. 100

LIGHT GREEN SF

1. Allmark, M.G., Grice, H.C., and Mannell, W.A. Chronic toxicity studies on food colors. II. Observations on the toxicity of FD and C green No. 2 (light green SF yellowish), FD and C orange No. 2 (orange SS), and FD and C red No. 32 (oil red XO) in rats. J. Pharm. Pharmacol., 8: 417-424, 1956.
2. Gangolli, et al., 1967, (see blue VRS, Ref. 6).
3. Gangolli et al., 1972 (see benzyl violet 4B, Ref. 4).
4. Gross, E., Über den Triphenylmethanfarbstoff Lichtgrun SF als Sarkomerreger bei der Ratte. Naunyn-Schmiedeberg's Arch. Exp. Path. Pharmak., 225: 175-179, 1955.
5. Gross, 1961 (see brilliant blue FCF. Ref. 8).
6. Grossmann, D.F., and Frey, J. Renal clearance of lissamine green in the rat. In: Peters, G., ed., Proceeding of a Symposium on Progress in Nephrology, 5th edition 1967, Berlin, Springer, pp. 391-394.
7. Hansen et al., 1966, (see fast green FCF, Ref. 4).
8. Harris, P.N. Production of sarcoma in rats with light green SF. Cancer Res., 7: 35-36, 1947.
9. Heller, J., and Horacek, V. The influence of lissamine green on reabsorption of electrolytes and water in rats. Pflügers Arch., 323: 27-33, 1971.
10. Hess and Fitzhugh, 1954, (see benzyl violet 4B, Ref. 6).
11. Hess and Fitzhugh, 1955, (see benzyl violet 4B, Ref. 7).
12. Hesselbach and O'Gara, 1960 (see fast green FCF, Ref. 8).
13. Hooson et al., 1973 (see blue VRS, Ref. 11).
14. Iga et al., 1971 (see brilliant blue FCF, Ref. 13).
15. Iga et al., 1971 (see brilliant blue FCF, Ref. 14).
16. Krauze, S., and Piekarski, L., Studies on affinity of dyes to animal tissue proteins. Part V. Light green SF yellowish bounding to tissue proteins of mice. Roczn. PZH., 15: 459-450, 1964.
17. Kugaczewska and Krauze, 1972 (see amaranth, Ref. 42).
18. Lu and Lavallée, 1964 (see benzyl violet 4B, Ref. 9).
19. Lynch, R.E., Schneider, E.G., Strandhoy, J.W., Willis, L.R., and Knox, F.G. Effect of lissamine green dye on renal sodium reabsorption in the dog. J. Appl. Physiol., 35: 169-171, 1973.
20. Nelson and Davidow, 1957 (see benzyl violet 4B, Ref. 13).
21. Nelson and Hagan, 1953 (see amaranth, Ref. 50).
22. Piekarski, L. Studies on the affinity of dyes to animal tissue proteins. II. Free and bound dyes after administration in diet. Roczn. PZH, 15: 389-395, 1964.
23. Piekarski, L. Studies on the affinity of dyes to animal tissue proteins. III. Free and bound dyes after subcutaneous administration. Roczn. PZH, 15: 397-404, 1964.
24. Schiller, W. Rat sarcoma produced by the injection of the dye, light green FS. Amer. J. Cancer, 31: 486-490, 1937.
25. Waterman and Lignac, 1958 (see chrysoine, Ref. 5).

LITHOL RUBINE BK

1. Acute oral administration to dogs of D and C Red No. 7, Red No. 19, Red No. 36, and Orange 17. Unpublished report from Hazleton Labs, 1961.
2. Durloo, R.S., and Woodard, G. Safety evaluation of D and C Red No. 7 in a teratology study in the rat. Unpublished report from Woodard Research Corporation, Herndon, Va. sumbitted to the Inter-Industry Color Committee, 1972.

3. Hansen et al., 1958 (see eosine, Ref. 6).
4. Report to TGA acute oral administration: rats. D and C Red 7, D and C Red 19, D and C Red 36, D and C Orange 17. Unpublished re-report from Hazelton Labs, 1961.
5. Safety evaluation of D and C Red No. 7: dermal toxicity in the rabbit. Unpublished report from Leberco Labs, 1962.
6. Subject left-time skin painting studies in mice with D and C Orange 17, D and C Red 7, D and C Red 9, D and C Red 10. Unpublished port from Leberco Labs, 1964.
7. Two-year feeding studies in rats with D and C Red 7, D and C Red 19, D and C Orange 17. Unpublished report from Hazleton Labs, 1964.
8. Weil, C.S., and Carpenter, C. Results of inclusion intthe diet of rats for three-generation. Unpublished report from Mellon Institute, Carnegie, Mellon University, Pittsburg, Pa., submitted to the Inter-Industry Color Committee by the Cosmetic, Toiletry and Fragrance Association, Inc., 1973.

LYCOPENE

1. Zbinden and Stder, 1958 (see annatto, Ref. 6).

MAGENTA

1. Bonser et al., 1956 (see auramine, Ref. 3).
2. Case and Pearson, 1954 (see auramine, Ref. 4).
3. Druckrey, H., Nieper, H.A., and Lo, H.W., Carcinogene Wirkung von Parafuchsin im Injektionsversuch an Ratten. Naturwissenschaften, 43: 543-544, 1956.
4. Hueper, W.C. Occupational Tumours and Allied Diseases, Springfield, Ill., Thomas Publishing Co., 1942.
5. Mannell et al., 1962 (see benzyl violet 4B, Ref. 10).
6. Nelson and Hagan, 1953 (see amaranth, Ref. 50).
7. Rehn, L. Blasengeschwulste bei Fuchsinarbeitern. Arch. klin. Chir., 50: 588, 1895.
8. Willheim and Ivy, 1953 (see acid fuchsine, Ref. 4).
9. Yoshida, T., Shimanchi, T., and Klin, C. Experimentelle Studien über die Entwicklung des Harnblasentumours. Gann, 35: 272-274, 1941.

MALACHITE GREEN

1. Allmark, M.G., Mannell, W.A., and Grice, H.C. Chronic toxicity on food colors. III. Observations on the toxicity of malachite green, new coccine, and nigrosine in rats. J. Pharm. Pharmacol. 9, 622-628.
2. Brock, N., and Erhardt, A. Zur Pharmakotherapie der Oxyuriasis. I. Pharmacologische, toxikologische, und chemotherapeutische Unter-suchungen mit Pararoasnilinfarbstoffen un ihren Carbinol basen. Arzneimittel-Forsch. 1: 5-21, 1951.
3. Deschiens, R., and Bablet, J. Recherches sur la toxicité des déri-vés triphénylméthanique anthelminthiques. C.R. des Séances de la Societé de Biologie, 138: 838-839, 1944.
4. Hecht, G. Unpublished results. Summary in Ref. 1 (acid fuchsine FB, p. 66).
5. Piekarski, 1964 (see light green SF, Ref. 22).
6. Piekarski, 1964 (see light green SF, Ref. 23).
7. Sikorska and Krauze, 1962 (see acid fuchsine FB, Ref. 3).

8. Werth, G., Die Erzeugung von Störungen im Erbgefüge und von Tumoren durch experimentelle Gewabsanoxie. *Arzneimittel-Forsch.* 8(12): 735, 1950.
9. Werth, G. Transplantationsergebnisse mit durch Malachitgrun erzeugten Tumoren. *Z. Krebsforsch.*, 64: 234-244, 1961.

METHANIL YELLOW

1. Cook et al., 1940 (see amaranth, Ref. 24).
2. Hecht, G. Unpublished results. Summary in Ref. 1 (acid fuchsine FB p. 22).
3. Kawai, 1928 (see auramine, Ref. 6).

METHYL VIOLET

1. Hecht, G. Unpublished results. Summary in Ref. 1 (acid fuchsine FB, p. 76).
2. Kawai, 1928 (see auramine, Ref. 6).
3. Schaeppi, H.U. Summary in Ref. 1 (acid fuchsine FB, p. 78).

NAPHTHOL BLUE BLACK

1. U.S. Food and Drug Administration, 1964 (see benzyl violet 4B, Ref. 1).

NAPHTHOL YELLOW S

1. Diemair and Hausser, 1951 (see brilliant black BN, Ref. 2).
2. Klinke, 1955 (see brilliant blue FCF, Ref. 15).
3. Nelson, A.A. and Fitzhugh, O.G. Mortality and ulcerovegetative intestinal lesions in rats from feeding naphthol yellow S (FD and C Yellow No. 1). *Fed. Proc.* 17, 449.
4. Waterman and Lignac, 1958 (see chrysoine, Ref. 5).

NIGROSINE

1. Allmark et al., 1957 (see malachite green, Ref. 1).
2. Hecht, G. Unpublished results. Summary in Ref. 1 (acid fuchsine FB, p. 99).
3. Waterman and Lignac, 1958 (see chrysoine, Ref. 5).

OIL ORANGE SS

1. Allmark et al., 1956 (see light green SF, Ref. 1).
2. Baer, R.L., Leider, M., and Mayer, R.L. Possible exzematous cross-hypersensitivity between paraphenylenediamine and azo-dyes certified for use in foods, drugs and cosmetics. *Proc. Soc. Exp. Biol.* (N.Y.), 67: 489-494, 1948.
3. Bonser, G.M., Clayson, D.B., and Jull, J.W. Induction of tumours with 1-(2-tolylazo)-2-naphthol (oil orange TX). *Nature (London)*, 174:879-880, 1954.
4. Bonser et al., 1956 (see auramine, Ref. 3).
5. Clayson, D.B., Jull, J.W., and Bonser, G.M. The testing of ortho-hydroxy-amines and related compounds by bladder implantation and a discussion of their structural requirements for carcinogenic activity. *Brit. J. Cancer*, 12: 222-230, 1958.

6. Climenko, D.R. Study of the toxicity of ortho-tolueno-azo-beta-naphthol, an oil soluble food dye. AMA Journal, 109: 493, 1937.
7. Fitzhugh, O.G., Nelson, A.A., and Bourke, A.R. Chronic toxicities of two food colors, FD and C Red No. 32 and FD and C Orange No. 2. Fed. Proc., 15: 422, 1956.
8. Nelson and Davidow, 1957 (see benzyl violet 4B, Ref. 13).
9. Radomski and Deichmann, 1956 (see amaranth, Ref. 54).
10. Toxicity studies on the rat with oil orange SS. Unpublished report from the Department of Pharmacology of the Japanese National Institute of Hygienic Sciences 1964.
11. U.S. Food and Drug Administration, Department of Health, Education and Welfare, Title 21, Food and Drugs, Part 135, Fed. Regis. 20: 8492, 1955.
12. Vos, B.T., Radomski, J.L., and Fuyat, H.N., Orange I. Cathartic actions of FD and C Orange I and other coal-tar food dyes. Fed. Proc., 12: 376.
13. Willheim and Ivy, 1953 (see acid fuchsine FB, Ref. 4).

OIL ORANGE XO

1. Allmark et al., 1956 (see light green SF, Ref. 1).
2. Baer et al., 1948 (see oil orange SS, Ref. 4).
3. Bonser et al., 1956 (see auramine, Ref. 3).
4. Carroll, R. Lesions of the liver produced by sudan dyes. J. Path. Bact., 87: 317-324, 1964.
5. Clayson et al., 1968 (see blue VRS, Ref. 2).
6. Fitzhugh et al., 1956 (see oil orange SS, Ref. 9).
7. Maruya, 1938 (see chrysoidine, Ref. 8).
8. Nelson and Davidow, 1957 (see benzyl violet 4B, Ref. 13).
9. Radomski, 1961 (see citrus red 2, Ref. 46).
10. Radomski, 1962 (see citrus red 2, Ref. 5).
11. Radomski and Deichmann, 1956 (see amaranth, Ref. 54).
12. Rofe, P. Azo dyes and Heinz bodies. Brit. J. Industr. Med., 14: 275-280, 1957.
13. U.S. Food and Drug Administration, 1955 (see oil orange SS, Ref. 2).
14. Vos et al., 1953 (see oil orange SS, Ref. 12).
15. Willheim and Ivy, 1953 (see acid fuchsine FB, Ref. 4).

OIL YELLOW AB

1. Acute toxicity in the mouse with oil yellow AB. Unpublished report from the Division of Pharmacology of the U.S. Food and Drug Administration, 1957.
2. Allmark, M.G., Grice, H.C., and Lu, F.C., Chronic toxicity studies in food colors. I. Observations on the toxicity of FD and C Yellow No. 3 (oil yellow AB) and FD and C Yellow No. 4 (oil yellow OB) in rats. J. Pharm. Pharmacol. 7: 591-603, 1955.
3. Badger, G.M., Cook, J.W., Hewett, C.L., Kennaway, E.L., Kennaway, N.M., and Martin, R.H. The production of cancer by pure hydrocarbons. Proc. Roy. Soc. B., 131: 170-182, 1942.
4. Baer et al., 1948 (see oil orange SS-Ref. 4).
5. Druckrey, H. Schädliche und unschädliche Farbstoffe fur Lebensmittel. Z. Krebsforsch., 60: 344-360, 1955.
6. Hansen, W.H., Fitzhugh, O.G., and Nelson, A.A. Chronic toxicities of two food colors: FD and C Yellow No. 3 and 4 (yellow AB and Yellow OB). Fed. Proc., 17: 375 (Abstract No. 1478), 1958.

7. Hansen, W.H., Nelson, A.A., and Fitzhugh, O.G. Chronic toxicity of yellow AB (1-phenylazo-2-naphthylamine) and yellow OB (1-O-toly-lazo-2-naphthylamine). Toxicol. Appl. Pharmacol., 5: 16-35, 1963.
8. Kozlov, I.N. Investigation of the biological effect of some synthetic dyes. Voprosy Pitaniya, 9(5): 41-48, 1940.
9. Nelson and Davidow, 1957 (see benzyl violet 4B, Ref. 13).
10. Radomski and Deichmann, 1956 (see amaranth, Ref. 54).
11. Rofe, 1957 (see oil orange XO, Ref. 13).
12. Salant, W. and Bengis, R. Physiological and pharmacological studies on coal-tar colors. I. Experiments with fat-soluble dyes. J. Biol. Chem., 27: 403-427, 1916.
13. Sugiura, K. Observations on rats fed with yellow AB. Proc. Soc. Exp. Biol. (N.Y.), 61: 301-302, 1946.
14. Vos et al., 1953 (see oil orange SS, Ref. 12).
15. Willheim and Ivy, 1953 (see acid fuchsine FB, Ref. 4).

OIL YELLOW OB

1. Allmark et al., 1955 (see oil yellow AB, Ref. 1).
2. Acute toxicity in the mouse with oil yellow AB. Unpublished report from the Division of Pharmacology of the U.S. Food and Drug Administration, 1957.
3. Badger et al., 1942 (see oil yellow AB, Ref. 3).
4. Hansen et al., 1958 (see oil yellow AB, Ref. 6).
5. Hansen et al., 1963 (see oil yellow AB, Ref. 7).
6. Kozlov, 1940 (see oil yellow AB, Ref. 8).
7. Ohtsuka, Y. Oral toxicity of oil soluble tar color oil yellow OB. Jap. J. Hyg. 23: 501-513, 1969.
8. Radomski and Deichmann, 1956 (see amaranth, Ref. 54).
9. Radomski, J.L., and Harrow, L.S. The metabolism of 1-(o-tolylazo)-2-naphthylamine (yellow OB) in rats. Industr. Med. Surg., 35: 882-888, 1966.
10. Rofe, 1957 (see oil orange XO, Ref. 13).
11. Salant and Bengis, 1916 (see oil yellow AB, Ref. 12).
12. Sugiura, K. Failure of yellow OB to produce neoplasma. Proc. Soc. Exp. Biol. Med., 50: 214-215, 1942.
13. Traub, E.F., Gordon, R.E., and van Dyke, L.S. Dermatitis from dyes and otherwise treated citrus fruits. J. Am. Med. Ass., 108: 872-874, 1937.
14. Vos et al., 1953 (see oil ora-ge SS, Ref. 12).
15. Willheim and Ivy, 1953 (see acid fuchsine FB, Ref. 4).

OLEORESIN OF PAPRIKA

1. Csedö, K. Studiul principilor active din ardeiul iute (Fructus capsici) indigen. Dissertation, University of Tirgu-mures, 1962.
2. Hoch-Ligéti, C. Production of liver tumours in rats by dietary means. Effect of feeding chili (Capsicum frutescens and anuum) to rats. Research communication to the V Cong. Int. Canc. p. 122, 1950.
3. Högyes, A. Beitrage zur physiologischen Wirkung der Bestandtheile des Capsicum annum (Spanischer Pfe fer). Arch. Exper. Path. Pharm. 9: 117-130, 1978.
4. Jancsó, N. Speicherung-Stoffanreicherung im Reticuloendothel und in der Niere. Verl. Akademiai Kiado (Budapest) 1955.
5. Molnár, J. Die pharmakologischen Wirkungen des Capsaicins des shaff-schmeckenden Wirkstoffes im Paprika. Arzneimittel-Forsch., 15: 718-727, 1965.

6. Pórszász, J., Such, G., and Pórszász-Gibiszer, K. Circulatory and respiratory chemoreflexes. I. Analysis of the site of action and receptor types of capsaicine. Acta Phys. Hung., 12: 189-205, 1957.
7. Toh, C.C., Lee, T.S., and Kiang, A.K. The pharmacological actions of capsaicin and analogues. Brit. J. Pharmacol., 10: 175-182, 1955.
8. Várady, M. and Koturnya, M. A paprika hatása (Die Wirkung des Paprikas). Preisaufgabe der medizinische Fakultät der Universität, Szeged, 1931.

ORANGE I

1. Baer et al., 1948 (see oil orange SS, Ref. 4).
2. Bourke, A.R., Nelson, A.A., and Fitahugh, O.G. Chronic toxicity of FD and C Orange No. 1, Fed. Proc., 15: 404, 1956.
3. Brown et al., 1977 (see cochineal/Carmine/carminic acid, Ref. 2).
4. Color certification. Miscellaneous Amendments. U.S. Food and Drug Administration, Dept. of Health, Education and Welfare, Title 21, Food and Drugs, Part 135, Federal Register, 20: 8492, 1955.
5. Cook et al., 1940 (see amaranth, Ref. 24).
6. Diemair and Hausser, 1951 (see brilliant black BN, Ref. 3).
7. Hallesy, D.W., and Doull, J. Acute and chronic toxicity of orange B and orange I in rats. J. Pharmacol. Exp. Ther., 116: 26 (Abstract), 1956.
8. Hecht, G., 1954. Unpublished results. Summary in Ref. 1 (acid fuchsine FB., p. 25).
9. Klinke, J. Unpublished results. Summary in Ref. 1 (acid fuchsine FB, p. 25).
10. Nelson and Davidow, 1957 (see benzyl violet 4B, Ref. 13).
11. Piekarski, 1964 (see light green SF, Ref. 22).
12. Radomski and Deichmann, 1956 (see amaranth, Ref. 54).
13. Sisley, P., and Porcher, C. Du sort de matières colorantes dans l'organisme animal. C.R. Acad. Sci. (Paris), 152: 1062-1064. 1911.
14. Summary of toxicity studies on colors: Orange I (FD and C Orange No. 1-No. 150). Unpublished report submitted to WHO by the U.S. Food and Drug Administration, 1964. Summary in WHO/FAO 1970, p. 47. (reported as US.. FDA, 1963).
15. Truhaut, R. Sur l'utilization des colorantes en thérapeutique et les dangers qui peuvent en résulter pour la snaté humaine. Chimie Moderne, 3: 337-350, 1958.
16. Vos et al., 1953 (see oil orange SS, Ref. 12).
17. Willheim and Ivy, 1953 (see acid fuchsine FB, Ref. 4).

ORANGE II

1. Cook et al., 1940 (see amaranth, Ref. 24).
2. Kawai, 1928 (see auramine, Ref. 6).
3. Piekarski, 1964 (see light green SF, Ref. 22).
4. Piekarski, 1964 (see light green SF, Ref. 23).

ORANGE G

1. Brantom, P.G., Gaunt, I.F., and Hardy, J. One-year toxicity study of orange G in the ferret. Fd. Cosmet. Toxicol. 15: 379-382, 1977.
2. Cook et al., 1940 (see amaranth, Ref. 24).
3. Daniel, 1962 (see erythrosine, Ref. 7).
4. Daniel, J.W. Enzymic reduction of azo food colourings. Fd. Cosmet. Toxicol., 5: 533-534, 1967.

5. Gaunt, I.F. Ph.D. Thesis. London University, 1973.
6. Gaunt, I.F., Wright, M., Grasso, P., and Gangolli, S.D., Short-term toxicity of orange G in rats. Fd. Cosmet. Toxicol., 9: 329-342, 1971.
7. Hansen et al., 1960 (see fluorescein, Ref. 3).
8. Long-term feeding studies on orange G in mice. Unpublished report from BIBRA, 1977.
9. Rofe, 1957 (see oil orange XO, Ref. 13).
10. Roxon et al., (see amaranth, Ref. 56).
11. Ryan et al., (see amaranth, Ref. 58).
12. Walker et al., 1972: unpublished results quoted in Fd. Cosmet. Toxicol., 11: 367-374, 1973.
13. Waterman and Lignac, 1958 (secchrysoine, Ref. 5).

ORANGE GGN

1. Bar and Griepentrog, 1960 (see amaranth, Ref. 14).
2. Eisenbrand, J., and Lang, E. Influence of azo dyes on acid production of lactic acid bacteria. V. Action of cleavage and air-oxidation products of brilliant black BN, crysoin, echtgelb extra, yellow 27175 N, yellow orange S, orange GGN, and tartrazine. Z. Lebensm.-Untersuch. U.-Forsch. 113: 48-52, 1960.
3. Galea et al., 1962 (see amaranth, Ref. 28).
4. Hecht, G. Unpublished results. See Ref. 1 (acid fuchsine FB, p. 32).
5. Hecht and Wingler, 1952 (see black 7989, Ref. 3).
6. Lang, 1967 (see brilliant black PN, Ref. 11).
7. Luck and Rickerl, 1960 (see amaranth, Ref. 45).
8. Ryan and Wright, 1961 (see amaranth, Ref. 59).
9. Sondergaard et al., 1977 (see allura red, Ref. 16).
10. Schormuller, J., and Schulz, W.B. Action of food colors on the succinic acid dehydrase and xanthine oxidase in vitro. Z. Lebensm.-Untersuch. U.-Forsch., 108: 9-17, 1958.
11. Sporn, M.P., and Gal'perin, S. Studies on the toxicity of chemicals added to food. Voprosy Pitaniya, 17: 48-53, 1958.
12. Sporn, A., and Heilpern, J. The toxicity of the orange GGN food folouring. Igiena, 7: 235-243, 1958.
13. Wingler, A., Dyes in foodstuff dyeing. The problem of exposure to cancer. 2. Krebsforsch. 59: 134-155, 1953.

ORANGE RN

1. Dacre, J.C. Acute and chronic toxicity studies on orange RN. Proc. Univ. Otaga Med. Sch., 47: 3-4, 1969.
2. Daniel, 1962 (see erythrosine, Ref. 7).
3. Gaunt, I.F., Brantom, P.G., Kiss, I.S., Grasso, P., and Gangolli, S.D. Short-term toxicity of orange RN in rats. Fd. Cosmet. Toxicol. 9: 619-630, 1971.
4. Hasselager, E., and Hansen, E. Peroral toxicity of orange RN in pigs: induction and reversibility of hepatic lesions. Abstract of data to be published 1977. Summary in WHO/FAO 1978a (to be issued).
5. Larsen, J.C., and Tarding, F. Studies on the metabolism of orange RN in the pig. Acta. Pharm. et toxicol. 39: 525-535, 1976.
6. Larsen, J.C., and Tarding, F. Studies on the absorption and excretion of ^{35}S-orange RN in rats and rabbits. Abstract of data presented at the 19th Meeting of the European Society of Toxicology, Copenhagen, June 19-22, 1977.

7. Olsen, P., and Hansen, E. Bile duct proliferation in pigs fed the food color orange RN. Acta. Pharm. Toxicol., 32: 314-316, 1973.
8. Olsen, P., Wurtzen, G., Hansen, E., Carstensen, J., and Poulsen, E. Short-term peroral toxicity of the food colour orange RN in pigs. Toxicology, 1: 249-260, 1973.
9. Walker, R. Intestinal degradation of azo food colours with particular reference to brown FK. Ph.D. Thesis, University of Reading, Reading, Berks, England., 1968.
10. Walker, 1970 (see azorubine, Ref. 22).
11. Wingler, 1953 (see orange GGN, Ref. 13).
12. Wurtzen, G., Larsen, J.C., and Tarding, F. Formation of methaemoglobin in vivo and in vitro after administration of orange RN. Scand. J. Clin. Lab. Invest. 29, Suppl. 126, 1972.

ORCHIL/ORCEIN

1. Truhaut, R. Resultats des experiences de toxicité à long terme effectuees avec deux colorants d'origine naturelle, le curcuma et l'orseille. C.R. 18ème Congrès de Sciences Pharmaceutiques. Bruxelles, 8-15 Septembre 1958.

PATENT BLUE V

1. Grasso and Golberg, 1966 (see blue VRS, Ref. 7).
2. Gangolli et al., 1967 (see blue VRS, Ref. 6).
3. Grasso et al., 1971 (see benzyl violet 4B, Ref. 3).
4. Kugaczewska and Krauze, 1972 (see amaranth, Ref. 42).
5. Truhaut, R. Additifs aux aliments: les risques de nocivité pouvant resulter de leur emploi inconsideré. Les méthods de prevention. R.C. Ist. Sup. Sanit., 25: 796-919, 1962.

PONCEAU 2R (MX)

1. Bonser et al., 1956 (see auramine, Ref. 3).
2. Cook et al., 1940 (see amaranth, Ref. 24).
3. Crampton, R.F., Gray, T.J.B., Grasso, P., and Parke, D.V. Long-term studies on chemically induced liver enlargement in the rat. II. Transient induction of microsomal enzymes leading to liver damage and nodular hyperplasia produced by safrole and ponceau MX. Toxicology, 7: 307-326, 1977.
4. Daniel, 1962 (see erythrosine, Ref. 7).
5. Grasso, P., and Gray, T.J.B. Long-term studies on chemically induced liver enlargement in the rat. III. Structure and behaviour of the hepatic nodular lesions induced by ponceau MX. Toxicology, 7: 327-347, 1977.
6. Grasso, P., Lansdown, A.B.G., Kiss, I.S., and Gaunt, I.F. Nodular hyperplasia in the rat liver following prolonged feeding with ponceau MX. Fd. Cosmet. Toxicol., 7: 425-442, 1969.
7. Hall, D.E., Lee, F.S., and Fairweather, F.A. Acute (mouse and rat) and short-term (rat) toxicity studies on ponceau MX. Fd. Cosmet. Toxicol., 4: 375-382, 1966.
8. Iga, T., Awazu, S., Hanano, M., and Nogami, H. Pharmacokinetic studies of biliary secretion. I. Comparison of the excretion behaviour in azo dyes and indigo carmine. Chem. Pharm. Bull., 18: 2431-2440, 1970.
9. Ikeda, Y. Long-term study of ponceau MX in rats and mice. Fd. Cosmet. Toxicol., 4: 361-363, 1966.

10. Ikeda, Y., Horiuchi, S., Furuya, T., and Omori, Y. Chronic toxicity of ponceau MX in the rat. Fd. Cosmet. Toxicol., 4: 485-492, 1966.
11. Ikeda, Y., Horiuchi, S., Kobayashi, K., Furuya, T., and Kohgo, K., Carcinogenicity of ponceau MX in the mouse. Fd. Cosmet. Toxicol. 6: 591-598, 1968.
12. Lindstrom, H.V. The metabolism of FD and C Red No. 1. I. The fate of 2,4-meta-xylidine in rats. Fed. Proc., 19: 183, 1960.
13. Rofe, 1957 (see oil orange XO, Ref. 13).
14. Ryan and Wright, 1961 (see amaranth, Ref. 59).
15. Sako et al., 1977 (see amaranth, Ref. 60).
16. Urakubo, G. Distribution (in experimental animals) and excretion of sulfur-35-labelled ponceau MX. Shokuhin Eiseigaku Zasshi, 8: 489-493, 1967.
17. Waterman and Lignac, 1958 (see chrysoine, Ref. 5).
18. Willheim and Ivy, 1953 (see acid fuchsine FB, Ref. 4).

PONCEAU 3R

1. Aiso, K., Kanisawa, M., Okamoto, T., and Chujo, T., Chronic oral toxicity and carcinogenicity of ponceu 3R. Shokuhin Eiseigaku Zasshi, 7: 211-221, 1966.
2. Aiso, K., et al., 1966.
3. Baer et al., 1948 (see oil orange SS, Ref. 4).
4. Bonser, G.M., Boyland, E., Busby, E.R., Clayson, D.B., Grover, P.L., and Jull, J.W. A further study of bladder implantation in the mouse as a means of detecting carcinogenic activity: use of crushed paraffin wax or stearic acid as the vehicle. Brit. J. Cancer, 17: 127-136, 1963.
5. Daniel, 1962 (see erythrosine, Ref. 7).
6. Graham and Allmark, 1959 (see amaranth, Ref. 32).
7. Grice, H.C., Mannell, W.A., and Allmark, M.G. Liver tumours in rats fed ponceau 3R. Toxicol. Appl. Pharmacol., 3: 509-520, 1961.
8. Hansen, W.H., Davis, K.J., Fitzhugh, O.G., and Nelson, A.A. Chronic oral toxicity of ponceau 3R. Toxicol. Appl. Pharmacol. 5: 105-118, 1963.
9. Kanisawa, M., Okamoto, T., Chujo, T., and Aiso, K. Histopathological observations in rats fed ponceau 3R (food red No. 1). Ann. Rep. Inst. Food Microbiol. Chiba Univ., 18: 45-54, 1965.
10. Lindstrom, 1960 (see ponceau 2R, Ref. 12).
11. Lindstrom, H.V. The metabolism of FD and C Red. No. 1. II. The fate of 2,6-metaxylidine in rats. Fed. Proc., 20: 243 (abstract).
12. Lindstrom, H.V., and Hansen, W.H. The metabolism of FD and C Red. No. 1. III. The fate of 2,5-paraxylidine in rats and the relation between toxicity and metabolism of xylidine isomers. Fed. Proc. 21: 450, (abstract).
13. Lindstrom, H.V., Hansen, W.H., Nelson, A.A., and Fitzhugh, O.G. The metabolism of FD and C Red. No. 1. II. The fate of 2,5-paraxylidine in rats and observations on the toxicity of xylidine isomers. J. Pharmacol. Exp. Ther., 142: 257-263, 1963.
14. Lindstrom, H.V., Wallace, W.C., Hansen, W.H., Nelson, A.A., The metabolism of FD and C Red. No. 1. IV. The metabolism and toxicity of pseudocumidine and mesidine in rats. Fed. Proc., 22: 188, 1963.
15. Mannell, W.E. Further investigations on the production of liver tumours in rats by ponceau 3R. Fd. Cosmet. Toxicol., 2: 169-174, 1964.
16. Morris, H.P., and Wagner, B.P. Development of "minimum deviation" hepatomas. In: Wolfson, K.G., ed., Proceedings of the VIIIth

International Cancer Congress, Moscow, 1962, Moscow, Medgiz, p. 143, 1962.

17. Sako et al., 1977 (see amaranth, Ref. 60).
18. Toxicity studies of metabolites of ponceau 3R. Fd. Cosmet. Toxicol., 2: 83-84, 1964.
19. Truhaut, 1962 (see patent blue V, Ref. 5).
20. Willheim and Ivy, 1953 (see acid fuchsine FB, Ref. 4).

PONCEAU 4R

1. Allmark et al., 1957 (see malachite green, Ref. 1).
2. Andrianova, 1970 (see amaranth, Ref. 3).
3. Amos and Drake, 1977 (see amaranth, Ref. 2).
4. Bär and Griepentrog, 1960 (see amaranth, Ref. 14).
5. Burnett, C.M. Teratogenic studies with certified colors in rats and rabbits. Inter-Industry Color Committee. Society of Toxicology 13th Meeting (Abstract), 1972.
6. Gaunt, I.F., Farmer, M., Grasso, P., and Gangolli, S.D. Acute (mouse and rat) and short-term (rat) toxicity studies on ponceau 4R. Fd. Cosmet. Toxicol., 5: 187-194, 1967.
7. Gaunt, I.F., Grasso, P., Creasey, M., and Gangolli, S.D. Short-term toxicity studies on ponceau 4R in the pig. Fd. Cosmet. Toxicol. 7: 443-449, 1969.
8. Gross, E. Unpublished results. Summary in Ref. 1 (acid fuchsine FB, p. 41).
9. Hecht, G. Unpublished results. Summary in Ref. 1 (acid fuchsine FB, p. 41).
10. Klinke, J. Unpublished results. Summary in Ref. 1 (acid fuchsine FB, p. 41).
11. Kugaczewska and Krauze, 1972 (see amaranth, Ref. 42).
12. Larsson, 1975 (see amaranth, Ref. 43).
13. Lück and Rickerl, 1960 (see amaranth, Ref. 45).
14. Mason, P.L., Gaunt, I.F., Butterworth, K.R., and Hardy, J. Long-term toxicity of ponceau 4R in mice. Unpublished report from the BIBRA (Research Report No. 1/1974) submitted to WHO, 1974. Summary in WHO/FAO 1978b (to be issued).
15. Meyer, O., and Hausen, E.V. A study of the embryotoxicity of the food color ponceau 4R in rats. Toxicology, 5(2): 201-207, 1975.
16. Pierce, E.C. Multigeneration reproduction studies with certified colors in rats. Inter-Industry Color Committee. Society of Toxicology 13th Annual Meeting, 1974.
17. Ryan and Wright, 1961 (see amaranth, Ref. 59).
18. Sako, 1977 (see amaranth, Ref. 60).
19. Sikorska and Krauze, 1962 (see acid fuchsine FB, Ref. 3).
20. Walker, 1968 (see orange RN, Ref. 10).
21. Holmberg, D. (see amaranth, Ref. 70).

PONCEAU 6R

1. Bär and Griepentrog, 1960 (see amaranth, Ref. 14).
2. Druckrey, H. Summary in Ref. 1 (acid fuchsine FB, p. 42).
3. Gross, E. Unpublished results. Summary in Ref. 1 (acid fuchsine FB, p. 42).
4. Hacht, G. Unpublished results. Summary in Ref. 1 (acid fuchsine FB, p. 42).
5. Lück and Rickerl, 1960 (see amaranth, Ref. 45).

6. Michaelsson and Juhlin, 1970 (see amaranth Ref. 49).
7. Sonderggard et al., 1977 (see allura red, Ref. 16).

PONCEUA SX

1. Andrianova, 1970 (see amaranth, Ref. 3).
2. Color additives. Color certification, FD and C No. 4. Fed. Reg., 29: 16983, 1964.
3. Davis, K.J., Nelson, A.A., Zwickey, R.E., Hansen, W.H., and Fitzhugh, O.G. Chronic toxicity of poceau SX to rats, mice and dogs. Toxicol. Appl. Pharmacol., 8: 306-317, 1966.
4. Graham and Allmark, 1959 (see amaranth, Ref. 32).
5. Iga et al., 1970 (see ponceau 2R, Ref. 8).
6. Lu and Lavallee, 1964 (see benzyl violet 4B, Ref. 9).
7. Radomski and Deichmann, 1956 (see amaranth, Ref. 54).
8. Radomski and Mellinger, 1962 (see amaranth, Ref. 55).
9. Roxon et al., 1967 (see amaranth, Ref. 56).
10. Ryan and Wright, 1961 (see amaranth, Ref. 59).
11. Ryan et al., 1968 (see amaranth, Ref. 58).
12. Vos et al., 1953 (see oil orange SS, Ref. 12).
13. Willheim and Ivy, 1953 (see acid fuchsine FB, Ref. 4).

QUERCITIN/QUERCITRON

1. Ambrose, A.M., Robbins, D.J., and De Eds, F. Comparative toxicities of quercitin and quercitron. J. Amer. Pharm. Assoc. Sci. Ed., 41: 119-122, 1952.
2. Booth, A.N., Murray, C.W., Jones, F.T., and De Eds, F. The metabolic fate of rutin and quercitin in the animal body. J. Biol. Chem., 223: 251-257, 1956.
3. Douglass, C.D., and Hogan, R. Formation of protocatechuic acid from quercitin by rat kidney in vitro. J. Biol. Chem., 230: 625-629, 1958.
4. Hardigree, A.A., and Epler, J.L., Eighth Annual Meeting, Environmental Mutagen Society, February 13-17, 1977. Colorado Springs, Colorado.
5. Kallianos, A.G., Petrakis, P.L., Shetlar, M.R., and Wender, S.H., Preliminary studies on degradation products of quercitin in the rat's gastrointestinal tract. Arch. Biochem., 81: 430-433, 1959.
6. Kato, H., Folia Pharm. Japan, 47: 93-102, 1951 (Chem. Abst. 46, No. 6749E, 1952).
7. Masri, M.S., Booth, A.N., and De Eds, F. The metabolism and acid degradation of quercitin. Arch. Biochem., 85: 284-286, 1959.
8. Murray, C.W., Booth, A.N., De Eds, F., and Jones, F.T. Absorption and metabolism of rutin and quercitin in the rabbit J. Amer. Pharm. Assoc. Sc. Ed., 43: 361-364, 1954.
9. Nakagawa, Y., Shetlar, M.R., and Wender, S.H. Cataract development in rats fed commercial quercitin. Proc. Soc. Exp. Biol., 108: 401-402, 1961.
10. Petrakis, P.L., Kallianos, A.G., Wender, S.H., and Shetlar, M.R., Metabolic studies of quercitin labelled with C^{14}. Arch. Biochem. 85: 264-271, 1959.
11. Stelzig, D.A., and Ribeiro, S. Proc. Soc. Exp. Biol. Med., 141: 346-349, 1972.

QUINOLINE YELLOW

1. Bär and Griepentrog, 1960 (see amaranth, Ref. 14).
2. Hansen et al., 1960 (see fluorescein, Ref. 3).
3. Lu and Lavallée, 1964 (see benzyl violet 4B, Ref. 9).
4. Luck and Reckerl, 1960 (see amaranth, Ref. 45).
5. Oettel et al., 1965(see indanthrene blue RS, Ref. 5).
6. Smith, J.M. Quinoline yellow. Segment II. Rabbit teratology study. Unpublished report from Bio-Dynamics, Inc., to the Inter-Industry Color Committee 1972. Summary in WHO/FAO 1975a, p. 28.
7. Smith, J.M., Wilson, N.W., Rosselet, C., Andresen, W., and Kasner, J.A. A three generation reproduction study with D and C Yellow 10 in rats. Unpublished report from Bio-Dynamics, Inc., East Millstone, N.J., to the Inter-Industry Color Committee 1973. Summary in WHO/ FAO 1975a, p. 28.

RED 10B

1. Daniel, 1962, (see erythrosine, Ref. 7).
2. Hansen, et al., 1960 (see fluorescein, Ref. 3).
3. Ryan and Wright, 1961 (see amaranth, Ref. 59).
4. U.S. Food and Drug Administration, 1964 (see benzyl violet 4B, Ref. 1).

RED 2G

1. Acute and short-term feeding studies on red G with associated haematological investigations. Unpublished report from the BIBRA (Research Report 3/1965) 1965. Summary in WHO/FAO 1978a (to be issued).
2. Acute toxicity by oral intubation, intraperitoneal injection of red 2G in several animal species. Summary of data from Unilever Ltd 1974. Summary in WHO/FAO 1978a (to be issued).
3. Daniel, J.W. The metabolism of azo dyes. V. Azo-geramine. Unpublished report from ICI, 1958. Summary in WHO/FAO 1978a (to be issued).
4. Daniel, 1962 (see erythrosine, Ref. 7).
5. Gellatly, J.B.M., and Burrough, R. Effect of diets containing aniline and metabolites of aniline on spleen weights; Pathology. Unpublished report from Unilever Ldt 1966. Summary in WHO/FAO 1978a (to be issued).
6. Gellatly, J.B.M., and Burrough, R. Pathology of red 2G and phenylhydroxylamine in rat diets. Unpublished report from Unilever, Ltd., 1967. Summary in WHO/FAO 1978a (to be issued).
7. Gellatly, J.B.M., Jenkins, F.P., Salmond, G., Robinson, J., and Marlow, K. Subacute toxicity of red 2G in mice. Unpublished report from Unilever Ltd., 1968. Summary in WHO/FAO 1978a (to be issued).
8. Jenkins, F.P., Campbell, P.J., Robinson, J., and Salmond, G. Metabolism of red 2g. Unpublished report from Unilever Ltd., 1966. Summary in WHO/FAO 1978a (to be issued).
9. Jenkins, F.P., Robinson, J., Gellantly, J.B.M., and Salmond, G. Effect of red 2G and phenylhydroxylamine on spleen weight. Unpublished report from Unilever Ltd., 1967. Summary in WHO/FAO 1978a (to be published).
10. Jenkins, F.P., Robinson, J., Gellantly, J.B.M., Salmond, G., and Campbell, P.J. Effect of diets containing aniline and metabolites of aniline on spleen weights. Unpublished report from Unilever Ltd., 1966. Summary in WEO/FAO 1978a (to be issued).

11. Jenkins, F.P., Salmond, G., and Gellantly, J.B.M. Subacute toxicity of red 2G in sausage meat, Unpublished report from Unilever Ltd., 1966. Summary in WHO/FAO 1978a (to be issued).
12. Jenkins, F.P., Salmond, G., Campbell, P.J., Hardy, J., and Robinson, J. Metabolism of red G by the rat liver homogenate. Unpublished report from Unilever Ltd., 1966. Summary in WHO/FAO 1978a (to be issued).
13. Jenkins, F.P., Salmond, G., Robinson, J., Campbell, P.J., and Gellantly, J.B.M. Subacute toxicity of red G. Unpublished report from unilever Ltd., 1966. Summary in WHO/FAO 1978a (to be issued).
14. Jenkins, F.P., Robinson, J., Salmond, G., andGroger, W., Chronic toxicity of red 2G: 80-week mouse feeding trial, living animals studies. Unpublished report from Unilever Ltd., 1971. Summary in WHO/FAO 1978a (to be issued).
15. Priestly, G., and O'Reilly, M.J. Protein binding and the excretion of some azo dyes in rat bile. J. Pharm. Pharmacol., 18: 41-45, 1966.
16. Parke, D.V. Studies in detoxification. The metabolism of 14C aniline in the rabbit and other animals. Biochem. J., 77: 494-503, 1960.
17. Robinson, J. Chronic toxicity of red 2G: 2-year rat feeding trial (0 and 0.5% red 2G), biochemical studies after feeding for 200 days. Unpublished report from Unilever Ltd., 1968. Summary in WHO/FAO 1978a (to be issued).
18. Robinson, J., and Paragreen, G. Reproduction in rats fed red 2G. Unpublished report from Unilever Ltd., 1971. Summary in WHO/FAO 1978a (to be issued).
19. Rofe, P. Induction of Heinz bodies by edible azo dyes. Unpublished report from ICI. Summary in WHO/FAO 1978a (to be issued).
20. Rofe, 1957 (see oil orange XO, Ref. 13).
21. Ryan and Wright, 1961 (see amaranth, Ref. 59).
22. Walker, R. Private communication to E.M. den Tonkelaar, National Institute of Public Health, Bilthoven, The Netherlands, 1971.

RESORCINE BROWN

1. U.S. Food and Drug Administration, 1964 (see benzyl violet 4B, Ref. 1).

RHODAMINE B

1. Bonser et al., 1956 (see auramine, Ref. 3).
2. Gangolli et al., 1972 (see benzyl violet 4B, Ref. 4).
3. Hansen et al., 1958 (see eosine, Ref. 6).
4. Kawai, 1928 (see auramine, Ref. 6).
5. Lück et al., 1963 (see eosine, Ref. 13).
6. Sikorska and Krauze, 1962 (see acid fuchsine FB, Ref. 3).
7. Umeda, 1956 (see eosine, Ref. 17).
8. U.S. Food and Drug Administration, 1964 (see benzyl violet 4B, Ref. 1).
9. Webb, J.M. Studies of the metabolism of rhodamine B (D and C Red 19). Fed. Proc., 19: 183, 1960.
10. Webb, J.M., and Hansen, W.H. Studies of the metabolism of rhodamine B. Toxicol. Appl. Pharmacol., 3: 86-95, 1961.
11. Webb, J.M., Hansen, W.H., Desmond, A., and Fitzhugh, O.G. Biochemical and toxicological studies of rhodamine B and 3,6-diaminofluoran. Toxicol. Appl. Pharmacol., 3: 696-706, 1961.
12. Willheim and Ivy, 1953 (see acid fuchsine FB, Ref. 4).

RHODAMINE 6G

1. Gangolli et al., 1972 (see benzyl violet 4B, Ref. 4).
2. Lück et al., 1963 (see eosine, Ref. 13).
3. Umeda, 1956 (see eosine, Ref. 17).

RIBOFLAVIN

1. Axelrod, A.E., Spies, T.D., and Elvehjem, C.A. Study of urinary riboflavin excretion in man. J. Clin. Invest., 20: 229-233, 1941.
2. Emmerie, A. On the state of urinary flavin excretion. Acta Brev. Neerl. Physiol., 8: 118, 1938.
3. Harrison, T.R. Principles of Internal Medicine, 4th Ed. New York: McGraw-Hill, 1962.
4. Khun, R., and Boulanger, P. Über die Giftigkeit der Flavine. Hoppe-Seylers Z. Physiol. Chem., 241: 233-238, 1936.
5. Koschara, W., Uber Harnlyochrome. Hoppe-Seylers Z. Physiol. Chem., 232: 101-116, 1935.
6. Levy, G., and Jusko, W.J. Factors affecting the absorption of ribo-flavin in man. J. Pharm. Sci., 55: 285-289, 1966.
7. Pellmont, B. Handbuch der Allgemeinen Pathologie, Band 11, p. 984, Berlin: Springer Verlag, 1962.
8. Recommended Dietary Allowances. Seventh Revision. A report of the Food and Nutrition Board, National Research Council. Pub. No. 1964 National Academy of Science, Washington, D.C., 1968.
9. Selye, H. The role played by the gastrointestinal tract in the absorption and excretion of riboflavin. J. Nutr., 25: 137-142, 1943.
10. Unna, K., and Greslin, J.G. Studies on the toxicity and pharmacology of riboflavin. J. Pharmacol. Exp. Ther., 76: 75-80, 1942.

SAFFRON/CROCIN/CROCITIN

1. Chang, P-Y., Wang, C.K., Liang, C.T., and Kuo, W. The pharmacological action of Zang Hong Hua (Crucus sativus L.). Effects on the uterus and estrous cycle. Yao Hsueh Hsueh Pao, 11: 94-100, 1964.
2. Frank, A. Auffallende Purpura bei artifiziellem Abort. Deut. Med. Wochschr., 86: 1618-1620, 1961.
3. Grisolia, S. Hypoxia, Saffron and cardiovascular disease. Lancet. 2: 41-42, 1974.

SCARLET GN

1. Bär and Griepentrog, 1960 (see amaranth, Ref. 14).
2. Hecht, G. Unpublished results. Summary in Ref. 1 (acid fuchsine FB, p. 34).
3. Lück and Rickerl, 1960 (see amaranth, Ref. 45).
4. Ryan and Wright, 1961 (see amaranth, Ref. 59).
5. Sikorska and Krauze, 1962 (see acid fuchsine FB, Ref. 3).
6. Sondergaard et al., 1977 (see allura red, Ref. 16).

SILVER

1. Anderson, W.A.D. In: Pathology, 1966. Saint Louis: C.V. Mosby, Vol. 1, 73.
2. Bader, K.F. Organ deposition of silver following silver nitrate therapy of burns. Fd. Cosmet. Toxicol. 5: 435, 1967.

3. Bala, Y., Liftshits, V.M., Plotko, S.A., Aksenov, G.I., and Kopy-
   lova, L.M. Age levels of trace elements in the human body. Voroneah.
   Gos. Med. Inst., 64: 37-44, 1969.
4. Bunyan, J., Diplock, A.I., Cawthorne, M.A., and Green, J. Vitamin
   E and stress. VIII. Nutritional effects of dietary stress with silver in vitamin E-deficient chicks and rats. Brit. J. Nutr., 22:
   165-182.
5. Chambers, J., Krieger, C.G., Kay, L., and Stroud, R. Silver ion inhibition of serine proteases. Crystallographic study of silver-
   trypsin. Biochem. Bioph. Res. Comm., 59: 70-74, 1974.
6. Deby, C., Bacq, Z.M., and Simon, D. In vitro inhibition of the bio-
   synthesis of a prostaglandin by gold and silver. Biochem. Pharm.,
   22: 3141-3143, 1973.
7. Furchner, J.E., Richmond, C.R., and Drake, G.A. Comparative metabolism of radionuclides in mammals. IV. Retention of silver 110-m
   in the mouse, rat, monkey and dog. Hlth. Phys., 15: 505-514, 1968.
8. Goldberg, A.A., Shapero, M., and Wilder, F. Antibacterial colloidal
   electrolytes: the potentiation of the activities of mercuric-,
   phenylmercuric- and silver ions by a colloidal sulphonic anion. J.
   Pharm. Pharmacol., 2: 20, 1949.
9. Goodman, L.S., and Gilman, A. The Pharmacological Basis of Thera-
   peutics. New York: McMillan, 3rd Ed., p. 965, 1965.
10. Grasso, P., Abraham, R., Hendy, R., Diplock, A.T., Golberg, L., and
    Green, J. The role of dietary silver in the production of liver
    necrosis in vitamin E-deficient rats. Exp. Mol. Pathol. 11: 186-
    199, 1969.
11. Ham, K.N., and Tange, J.D. Silver deposition in rat glomerular mem-
    brane. Aust. J. Biol. Med. Sci., 50: 423-434, 1972.
12. Hamilton, E.I., Minski, M.J., and Cleary, J.J. The concentration and
    distribution of some stable elements in healthy human tissues in the
    United Kingdom. Sci. Tot. Environm., 1: 341-374, 1972.
13. Hill, C.H., and Matrone, G. Chemical parameters in the study of in
    vitro and in vivo interactions of transition elements. Fed. Proc.,
    29: 1474-1481, 1970.
14. Hill, W.R., and Pillsbury, D.M., Argyria, the Pharmacology of Silver.
    Baltimore, Maryland: The Williams and Wilkins Co., 1939.
15. Hoey, M.J. The effects of metallic salts on the histology and func-
    tioning of the rat testes. J. Reprod. Fert., 12: 461-472, 1966.
16. Kent, N.L., and McCance, R.A. The absorption and excretion of minor
    elements by man. I. Silver, gold, lithium, boron, and vanadium.
    Bioch. J., 35: 837, 1941.
17. Kharchenko, P.D., Berdyshew, G.D., Stepanenko, P.Z., and Velikoivan-
    enko, A.A. Change in nucleic acid level in rat brain and liver dur-
    ing long-term introduction of silver ions in drinking water. Fiziol.
    Zh. (Kiev), 19: 362-368, 1973.
18. Jensen, L.S., Peterson, R.P., and Falen, L. Inducement of enlarged
    heart and muscular dystrophy in turkey poults with dietary silver.
    Poultry Sci., 53:57-64, 1974.
19. Nakamura, S., and Ogura, Y. Mode of inhibition of glucose oxidase
    by metal ions. J. Biochem. (Tokyo), 64: 439-447, 1968.
20. Nishioka, H. Mutagenic activities of metal compounds in bacteria.
    Mut. Res., 31: 185-189, 1975.
21. Oppenheimer, B.S., Oppenheimer, E.I., Danishefsky, I., and Stout.
    A.P., Carcinogenic effect of metals in rodents. Cancer Res. 16: 439-
    441, 1956.
22. Petering, 1976 (see gold, Ref. 5).

23. Peterson, R.P., Jensen, L.S., and Harrison, P.C. Effect of silver induced enlarged hearts during the first four weeks of life on subsequent performance of turkeys. Avian Dis., 17: 802-806, 1973.
24. Rich, L.L., Fpinette, W.W., and Nasser, W.K. Argyria presenting as cyanatic heart disease. Am. J. Cardiol., 30: 290-292, 1972.
25. Shouse, S.S., and Whipple, G.H., I. Effects of intravenous injection of colloidal silver upon the hematopoietic system in dogs. J. Exp. Med., 53: 413, 1931.
26. Swanson, A.B., Wagner, P.A., Ganther, H.E., and Hoekstra, W.G. Antagonistic effects of silver and tri-o-cresylphosphate on selenium and glutathione peroxidase in rat liver and erythrocytes. Fed. Proc., 33: 639, 1947.
27. Tripton, I.H., and Cook, M.J. Trace elements in human tissues. II. Adult subjects from the Unites States. Hlth. Phys., 9: 103-145, 1963.
28. Wagner, P.A., Hoekstra, W.G., and Ganther, H.E. Alleviation of silver toxicity by selenite in the rat in relation to tissue clutathione peroxidase. Proc. Soc. Exp. Biol. Med., 148: 1106-1110, 1975.
29. Wahlberg, J.E. Percutaneous toxicity of metal compounds. Arch. Environ. Health, 11: 201-204, 1965.
30. Winge, D.R., Premakumar, R., and Kajagopalan, K.V. Metal induced formation of metallothionein in rat liver. Arch. Biochem. Biophys. 170: 242 -252, 1975.

SUDAN I

1. Bonser, G.M. The experimental induction of cancer of the bladder. Acta Un. Int. Cancr., 18: 538-544, 1962.
2. Bonser, G.M., Bradshaw, L., Clayson, D.B., and Jull, J.M. A further study of the carcinogenic properties of ortho hydroxy-amines and related compounds by bladder implantation in the mouse. Brit. J. Cancer, 10: 539-546, 1956.
3. Bonser, G.M., Clayson, D.B., and Jull, J.W. The potency of 20-methyl cholanthrene relative to other carcinogens on bladder implantation. Brit. J. Cancer, 17: 235-241, 1963.
4. Childs, J.J., and Clayson, D.B. The metabolism of 1-phenylazo-2-naphthol in the rabbit. Biochem. Pharmacol., 15: 1247-1258, 1966.
5. Childs. J.J., Nakajima, C., and Clayson, D.B. The metabolsim of 1-phenyl-azo-2-naphthol in the rat with reference to the action of the intestinal flora. Biochem. Pharmacol., 16: 1555-1561, 1967.
6. Clayson, D.B., and Bonser, G.M. The induction of tumours of the mouse bladder epithelium by 4-ethylsulphonaphthalene-1-sulphonamide. Brit. J. Cancer, 19: 311-316, 1965.
7. Clayson, D.B., Lawson, T.A., Santana, S., and Bonser, G.M. Correlation between the chemical induction of hyperplasia and of malignancy in the bladder epithelium. Brit. J. Cancer, 19: 297-310, 1965.
8. Clayson, et al., 1968 (see blue VRS, Ref. 2).
9. Daniel, 1962 (see erythrosine, Ref. 7).
10. Hackmann, C., Untersuchungen uber die cancerogene Wirkung einiger fettloslicher Azofarbstoffe. Z. Krebsforsch., 57: 530-541, 1951.
11. Kirby, A.H.M., and Peacock, P.R. Liver tumours in mice injected with commercial food dyes. Glasgow Med. J., 30: 364-372, 1949.
12. Maruya, 1938 (see chrysoidine, Ref. 8).
13. Truhaut, 1958 (see orange I, Ref. 15).

SUDAN III

1. Carroll, 1964 (see oil orange XO, Ref. 5).
2. Conney, A.H., and Levin, W. Induction of hepatic 7,12-dimethyl-benz(a)-anthracene metabolism by polycyclic aromatic hydrocarbons and aromatic derivatives. Life Sci., 5: 465-471, 1966.
3. Huggins, C., and Paraki, J. Aromatic azo derivatives preventing mammary cancer and adrenal injury from 7,12-dimethylbenz(a) an-thracene. Proc. Nat. Acad. Sci., 53: 791-796, 1965.
4. Levin, W., and Conney, A.H. Stimulatory effect of polycyclic hydro-carbons and aromatic azo derivatives on the metabolism of 7,12-dimethylbenz(a)anthracene. Cancer Res., 27: 1931-1938.
5. Maruya, 1938 (see chrysoidine, Ref. 8).
6. Ryan, A.J., and Welling, P.G. Some observations on the metabolism and excretion of the bisazo dyes Sudan III and Sudan IV. Fd. Cosmet. Toxicol., 5: 755-761, 1967.
7. Salant and Bengis, 1916 (see oil yellow AB, Ref. 12).
8. Shear, M.J., and Stewart, H.L., 1941, In: Hartwell, J.L. Survey of Compounds Which Have Been Tested for Carcinogenic Activity, Washington, D.C., U.S. Government Printing Office (Public Health Service Publication No. 149).
9. Summary of toxicity studies on colors: D and C Red. 17. Unpublished report from U.S. Food and Drug Administration, 1964.
10. Waterman and Lignac, 1958 (see chrysoine, Ref. 5).
11. Wheatley, D.N., and Sims, P. Comparison of the efficacy of pre-treatment protection against adrenal necrosis induced by 7-hydroxy-methyl-12-methylbenz(a)anthracene and by 7-methyl-12-methyl-benz(a)anthracene in rats. Biochem. Pharmacol., 18: 2583-2587, 1969.
12. Willheim and Ivy, 1953 (acid fuchsine FB, Ref. 4).
13. Young, J.S. The experimental production of metaplasia and hyper-plasia in the serousal endothelium and of hyperplasia in the alveo-lar epithelium of the lung of the rabbit. J. Path. Bact., 31: 265-275, 1928.

SUDAN IV

1. Blacow, N.W. Ed. (1972) Martindale, The Extra Pharmacopoeia, 26th ed., London: The Pharmaceutical Press, p. 208.
2. Bullock, F.D., and Rohdenburg, G.L. Experimental "carcinomata" of animals and their relation to true malignant tumours. J. Cancer Res. 3: 227-273, 1918.
3. Echert, C.T., Cooper, Z.K., and Seelig, M.G. Scarlet red as a pos-sible carcinogenic agent. Arch. Path., 19: 83-90, 1935.
4. Fische-, B. Die experimentelle Erzeugung atypischer Epithelwucher-ungen und die Entstehung bösartiger Geschwülste. Münch. Med. Wschr. 53:2041-2047, 1906.
5. Hachmann, 1951 (see sudan I, Ref. 10).
6. Huguenin, B. Contribution à l'étude des hétérotopies épithéliales actives non carcinomateuses spontanées et expérimentales. Arch. Med. Exp., 22: 422-432, 1910.
7. Jores, L. Über Art und Zustandekommen der von B. Fischer mittels "Scharlachöl" erzeugten Epithelwucherungen. Münch. Med. Wschr., 54: 879-881, 1907.
8. Levin and Conney, 1967 (see sudan III, Ref. 5).
9. Meyer, A.W. Experimentelle Epithelwucherungen. Beitr. Path. Anat., 46: 437 451, 1909.

10. Podilchak, M. Cancerogensis and chronic inflammation. Acta. Biol. Med. Germ., 8:559-572, 1962.
11. Ryan and Welling, 1967 (see sudan III, Ref. 7).
12. Takeuchi, M. Über die Veränderungen der Milchdrüse der Maus nach Scharlachrotolivenölinjektion. Mitt Med. Fak. Kais, Univ. Tokyo, 20: 47-60, 1918.
13. Umeda, M. Production of rat sarcoma by injection of Tween 80 solution of scarlet red. Gann, 48: 579-580, 1957.
14. Umeda, M. Production of rat sarcoma by injection of Tween 80 solution of scarlet red. Gann, 49: 27-31, 1958.
15. Vasiliev, J.M., and Cheung, A.B. Evolution of epithelial proliferation induced by scarlet red in the skin of normal and carcinogen-treated rabbits. Brit. J. Cancer, 16: 238-245, 1962.
16. Willheim and Ivy, 1953 (see acid fuchsine FB, Ref. 4).
17. Waterman and Lignac, 1958 (see chrysoine, Ref. 5).

SUDAN G

1. Druckrey, 1955 (see chrysoin SGX "specially   pure," Ref. 1).
2. Druckrey, H. and Schmahl, D. Naturwissenschaften, 42: 215, 1955.
3. Farbwerke Hoechst, A.G., 1964 (see alkali blue, Fef. 1).
4. Hecht, G. Unpublished results. Summary in Ref. 1 (acid fuchsine FB, p. 5).
5. Kugaczewska and Krauze, 1972 (see amaranth, Ref. 42).
6. Waterman and Lignac, 1958 (see chrysoine, Ref. 5).

SUDAN RED G

1. Druckrey, 1955 (see chrysoin SGX "specially pure," Ref. 1).
2. Farbwerke Hoechst, A.G., 1964 (see alkali blue, Ref. 1).
3. Hecht, G. Unpublished results. Summary in Ref. 1 (acid fuchsine FB, p. 21).

SUNSET YELLOW FCF

1. Bär and Griepentrog, 1960 (see amaranth, Ref. 14).
2. Baer et al., 1948 (see oil orange SS, Ref. 4).
3. Bonser et al., 1956 (see auramine, Ref. 3).
4. Daniel, 1962 (see erythrosine, Ref. 7).
5. Despopoulos, 1968 (see amaranth, Ref. 25).
6. Gangolli et al., 1972 (see benzyl violet 4B, Ref. 4).
7. Gaunt, I.F., Farmer, M., Grasso, P., and Gangolli, S.D. Acute (rat and mouse) and short-term (rat) toxicity studies on sunset yellow FCF. Fd. Cosmet. Toxicol., 5: 747-754, 1967.
8. Gaunt, I.F., Kiss, I.S., Grasso, P., and Gangolli, S.D. Short-term toxicity study on sunset yellow FCF in the miniature pig. Fd. Cosmet. Toxicol. 7:9-16, 1969.
9. Gaunt, I.F., Manson, P.L., Grasso, P., and Kiss, I.S. Long-term toxicity of sunset yellow FCF in mice. Fd. Cosmet. Toxicol., 12: 1-10, 1974.
10. Graham and Allmark, 1959 (see amaranth, Ref. 32).
11. Kanisawa, M., Okamoto, T., Chujo, T., and Aiso, K. Chronic oral toxicity of sunset yellow FCF. Ann. Rep. Inst. Food Microbiol. Chiba Univ., 20: 101-110, 1967.
12. Kugaczewska and Krauze, 1972 (see amaranth, Ref. 42).
13. Lang, 1967 (see brilliant black BN, Ref. 11).
14. Lu and Lavallée, 1964 (benzyl violet 4B, Ref. 9).

15. Lück and Rickerl, 1960 (see amaranth, Ref. 45).
16. Manchon, Ph. and Lowy, R. Effet "pseudo-vitaminique" du Jaune Soleil sur la croissance du rat. Fd. Cosmet. Toxicol. 2: 453-456, 1964.
17. Mannell et al., 1958 (see amaranth, Ref. 47).
18. Oettel et al., 1965 (see indanthrene blue RS, Ref. 5).
19. Radomski and Mellinger, 1962 (see amaranth, Ref. 55).
20. Roxon et al.,1967 (see amaranth, Ref. 56).
21. Ryan et al., 1968 (see amaranth, Ref. 58).
22. Ryan and Wright, 1961 (see amaranth, Ref. 59).
23. Sako, et al., 1977 (see amaranth, Ref. 60).
24. Sikorska and Krauze, 1962 (see acid fuchsine FB, Ref. 3).
25. Summary of toxicity data on colours: FD and C Yellow No. 6. Unpublished report from the U.S. Food and Drug Administration 1964. Summary in WHO/FAO 1966, p. 85-86.
26. Sysoev, A.B. and Zhurkov, V.S. A study of the mutagenic activity of synthetic food dyes—sun yellow sunset FCF and its analogous compound—sun yellow K. Gig. I. Sanit. 9: 26-30, 1974.
27. Truhaut and Ferrando, 1975 (see amaranth, Ref. 67).
28. Willheim and Ivy, 1953 (see acid fuchsine FB, Ref. 4).

TARTRAZINE

1. Allan, A.J., and Roxon, J.J. Metabolism by intestinal bacteria: the effects of bile salts in tartrazine azo reduction. Xenobiotica, 4: 637, 1974.
2. Bär and Griepentrog, 1960 (see amaranth, Ref. 14).
3. Bertagni, P., Hiron, P.C., Millburn, P., Osiyemi, F.O., Smith, R.L. Turbert, H.B., and Williams, R.T. Sex and species difference in biliary excretion of tartrazine and lissamine fast yellow in the rat, guinea pig, and rabbit. The influence of sex hormones on tartrazine excretion in the rat. J. Pharm. Pharmac., 24(8): 620-624, 1972.
4. Daniel, 1962 (see erythrosine, Ref. 7).
5. Daniel, J.W. The in vivo absorption of organic electrolytes. Unpublished report from ICI, 1966.
6. Davies, K.J., Fitzhugh, O.G., and Nelson, A.A. Chronic rat and dog toxicity studies on tartrazine. Toxicol. Appl. Pharmacol. 6: 621-626, 1964.
7. Dept. of Pharmacology, Japanese National Institute of Hygienic Sciences. Unpublished report, 1969. Summary in WHO/FAO 1966, p. 90.
8. Despopoulos, 1968 (see amaranth, Ref. 25).
9. Diemair and Hausser, 1951 (see brilliant black PN, Ref. 3).
10. Graham and Allmark, 1959 (see amaranth, Ref. 32).
11. Hecht, G. Unpublished results. Summary in Ref. 1 (acid fuchsine FB, p. 64).
12. Ingram, A.J., Kiss, I.S., Gaunt, I.F., Grasso, P., and Butterworth, K.R. Long-term study on tartrazine in mice. Quoted in: Toxicology, 5: 3-42, 1975.
13. Klinke, J. Unpublished results. Summary in Ref. 1 (acid fuchsine FB, p. 64).
14. Kugaczewska and Krauze, 1972 (see amaranth, Ref. 42).
15. Jones, R., Ryan, A.J., and Wright, S.E. The metabolism and excretion of tartrazine in the rat, rabbit and man. Fd. Cosmet. Toxicol. 2: 447-452, 1964.
16. Lück and Rickerl, (see amaranth, Ref. 45).
17. Mannell et al., 1958 (see amaranth, Ref. 47).

18. Nelson and Hagan, 1953 (see amaranth, Ref. 50).
19. Roxon, J.J., Ryan, A.J., and Wright, S.E. Reduction of tartrazine by a _Proteus_ species isolated from rats. Fd. Cosmet. Toxicol., 4: 419-426, 1966.
20. Ryan and Wright, 1961 (see amaranth, Ref. 59).
21. Ryan, A.J., and Wright, S.E. Biliary excretion of some azo dyes related to tartrazine. Nature, 195: 1009, 1962.
22. Sako, 1977 (see amaranth, Ref. 60).
23. Sikorska and Krauze, 1962 (see acid fuchsine FB, Ref. 3).
24. Smith, J., Wilson, N.H., Rosselet, C., Andresen, W., and Kasner, J.A. A three generation reproduction study in rats with FD and C Yellow 5 (tartrazine) and teratological studies in the rabbit. Unpublished report from Bio-Dynamics, Inc. East Millstone, N.J., submitted to the Cosmetic, Toiletry and Fragrance Association, Inc. Quoted in Toxicology, 5: 3-42, 1975.
25. Waterman and Lignac, 1958 (see chrysoine, Ref. 5).
26. Willheim and Ivy, 1953 (see acid fuchsine, Ref. 4).
27. Wright, S.E., Aust. Fed. Manuf., 32 (7): 1963. Quoted in Bibra Bull. 298), 514, 1963.
28. Westöo, 1965 (see yellow 2G, Ref. 12).

THIAZINE BROWN R

1. Gross, E. Unpublished results. Summary in Ref. 1 (acid fuchsine FB, p. 60).
2. Hecht, G. Unpublished results. Summary in Ref. 1 (acid fuchsine FB, p. 60).

TITANIUM DIOXIDE

1. Brown, J.R., and Mastromatteo, E. Acute oral and parenteral toxicity of four titanate compounds in the rat. Industr. Med. Surg., 31: 302-304, 1962.
2. Fournier, P., De l'emploi de l'oxyde de titane pour l'étude quantitative de l'absorption intestinale. C.R. Acad. Sci. (Paris), 231: 1343-1344, 1950.
3. Isaac, and Ferch, 1976 (see aluminium, Ref. 17).
4. Lehman, K.B., and Herget, L. Studien über die hygienischen Eigenschaften des Titandioxyds und Titanweiss. Chem Ztg., 51: 793, 1927.
5. Lloyd, L.E., Rutherford, B.E., and Crampton, E.W. A comparison of titanium oxide and chronic oxide as index materials for determining apparent digestibility. J. Nutr., 56: 265-271, 1955.
6. Vernetti-Blina, L. Ricerche cliniche e sperimentali sull'ossido di titanio. Rif. Med., 47: 1516, 1928.
7. West, B., and Wyzan, H. Investigations of the possible absorption of titanium dioxide from the gastrointestinal tract. Unpublished report from the Central Medical Dept. of American Cyanamid Co., Wayne, N.J. Summary in WHO/FAO 1970, p. 55.

TURMERIC/CURCUMIN

1. Abraham, S., Abraham, S.K., and Radhamany, G. Mutagenic potential of the condiments; ginger, and turmeric. Cytologia, 41: 591-595, 1976.
2. Goodpasture, C.E., and Arrighi, F.E. Effects of food seasonings on cell cycle and chromosome morphology of mammalian cells in vitro with special reference to turmeric. Fd. Cosmet. Toxicol. 14: 9-14, 1976.

3. Rao, D.S., Sekhara, N.C., Satyanarayana, M.N., and Srinivasan, M. Effect of curcumin on serum and liver cholesterol levels in the rat. J. Nutr. 100: 1307-1315, 1970.
4. Sharma, O.P. Antioxidant activity of curcumin and related compounds. Biochem. Pharmacol.,25: 1811-1812, 1976.
5. Screenivasa, M. On going studies (short-term in rats, dogs, and monkeys, long-term studies in rats, and reproduction studies in rats). Central Food Technology Research Institute, Mysore, India. 1977.
6. Truhaut, 1958 (see orchil/orcein, Ref. 1).

ULTRAMARINES

1. Acute oral toxicity of 22 compounds in the male albino rats. Unpublished report from the International Research and Development Corporation, 1970.
2. Burakova, A.I., and Boiko, A.P. Ultramarine poisoning, Sud. Med. Ekspert, Kriminal. Sluzhbe Sledstviya, 5: 573-574, 1967.
3. Dunner, L., and Bagnall, D.J.T. Occupational lung disease and tuberculosis in ultramarine workers. Ind. Med. Surg., 24: 477-480, 1955.
4. Gurvich, V.N., Human toxicology in the professional production of dyestuffs. Proceedings of the First Republic Conference on Preventive Hygiene, 1926. Quoted in Vopr. Pit., 32(5): 52-58, 1973.
5. Large, E.W. "Hygienic Evaluation of Synthetic Food Dyes - A Review of the Literature." Amer. Perf. Cosmet. J., 77: 43, 1962.
6. Petrov, I.M. Toxicology of ultramarine administered by intramuscular injection. Publication from the Scientific Section of the Leningrad District. Quoted in Vopr. Pit., 32(5): 52-58, 1973.
7. Phillips, I., and Marks, G.C. British Plastics, 34: 386, 1961.
8. Volkova, N.A. Kunjev, V.V., and Popov, V.I., Material from the 17th Scientific Session of the Food Institute, AMN, Moscow, 1971, p. 43. Quoted in Vopr. Pit., 32(5): 52-58, 1973.
9. Volkova, N.A., Popov, V.I., and Sysoev, A.B. Hygienic evaluation of synthetic Food dyes. A review of the literature. Vopr. Pit., 32: 52-58, 1973.
10. Ward, R.J., Amos, C.C., Dawes, R.L.F. Man, V., and Preece, J.J. Ultramarine as a foodstuff pigment. Teratological studies. Unpublished report No. 1176 from Reckitt and Sons Ltd., Hull, England, 1966.
11. Ward, R.J., Cork, W.B., McCoubrey, A., Daves, R.L.F., and Somers, C.F. Analytical and toxicological study of ultramarine blue, RS-5. Unpublished report from Reckitt and Sons Ltd. Hull. England, (report No. 975), 1965.
12. Ward, R.J., Dawes, R.L.F., Preece, J.J., Inman, V., and Amos, C.C. Etude teratologique pour l'utilization de bleu d'outremer comme colorant alimentaire. Unpublished report from Reckitt and Sons Ltd., Hull, England, 1966.

VIOLAMINE R

1. Umeda, 1956 (see eosine, Ref. 17).

VIOLET 5BN

1. Miller and Pybus, 1954 (see blue VRS, Ref. 14).

WATER BLUE I

1. Farbwerke Hoechst, 1964 (see alkali blue, Ref. 1).

XANTHOPHYLLS

1. Antener, J., Neuweiler, W., Althaus, U., and Richter, R.H.H., Int. Z. Vitamin-Forsch., 32: 459, 1962.

YELLOW 2 G

1. Bertagni et al., 1972 (see tartrazine, Ref. 4).
2. Evans, J.G., Gaunt, I.F., Kiss, I.S., and Butterworth, K.R. Long-term toxicity of yellow 2G in mice. Unpublished report from BIBRA (Research Report No. 13/1975), 1975. Summary in WHO/FAO 1978a (to be issued).
3. Gaunt, I.F., Butterworth, K.R., Grasso, P., and Hooson, J., A short-term toxicity feeding study of yellow 2G in pigs. Fd. Cosmet. Toxicol., 13: 1-5, 1975.
4. Gaunt, I.F., Carpanini, F.M.B., Kiss, I.S., and Grasso, P., Short-term toxicity of yellow 2G in rats. Fd. Cosmet. Toxicol., 9, 343-353, 1971.
5. Hooson, J., Gaunt, I.F., Hardy, J., Gangolli, S.D., and Butterworth, K.R. Long-term toxicity study of yellow 2G in the rat. Unpublished report from BIBRA (Research Report No. 18/1975), 1975. Summary in WHO/FAO 1978a (to be issued).
6. Priestly and O'Reilly, 1966. (see red 2G, Ref. 15).
7. Roxon, et al., 1967 (see amaranth, Ref. 56).
8. Ryan et al., 1968 (see amaranth, Ref. 58).
9. Ryan and Wright, 1961 (see amaranth, Ref. 59).
10. Ryan and Wright, 1962 (see tartrazine, Ref. 21).
11. Walker, 1970 (see azorubine, Ref. 22).
12. Westöo, G. On the metabolism of tartrazine in the rat. Acta Chem. Scand., 19: 1309, 1965.

YELLOW 27175 N

1. Bär and Griepentrog, 1950 (see amaranth, Ref. 14).
2. Hecht, G. Unpublished results. Summary in Ref. 1 (acid fuchsine FB, p. 30).

WHO/FAO REFERENCES

WHO/FAO 1966. Specifications for identity and purity, and toxicological evaluation of food colours. FAO Nutrition Meetings Report Series No. 38B; WHO/Food Add./66: 25, 1966.
WHO/FAO 1970. Toxicological evaluation of some food colours, etc. FAO Nutrition Meetings Report Series No. 46A; WHO/Food Add./70: 36, 1970.
WHO/FAO 1971. Toxicological evaluation of some extraction solvents and certain other substances. FAO Nutrition Meetings Report Series No. 48A; WHO/Food Add./70: 39, 1971.
WHO/FAO 1972a. Toxicological evaluation of some enzymes, modified starches and certain other substances. FAO Nutrition Meetings Report Series No. 50A; WHO Food Additives Series No. 1, 1972.
WHO/FAO 1972b. Evaluation of mercury, lead, cadmium and the food additives amaranth, diethylpyrocarbonate and octyl gallate. FAO Nutrition Meetings Report Series No. 51A; WHO Food Additives Series No. 4, 1972.
WHO/FAO 1975a. Toxicological evaluation of some food colours, etc. FAO Nutrition Meetings Report Series No. 55A; WHO Food Additives Series No. 8, 1975.

WHO/FAO 1975b. Toxicological evaluation of some food colours, etc. FAO
Nutrition Meetings Report Series No. 55 (54A) WHO Food Additives
Series No. 6, 1975.